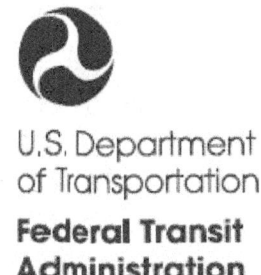

U.S. Department
of Transportation
**Federal Transit
Administration**

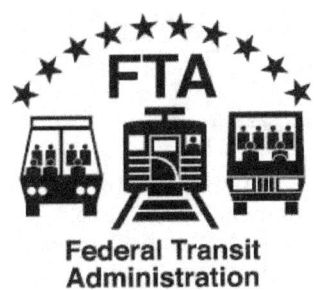

Federal Transit
Administration

Optimization Models for Prioritizing Bus Stop Facility Investments for Riders with Disabilities

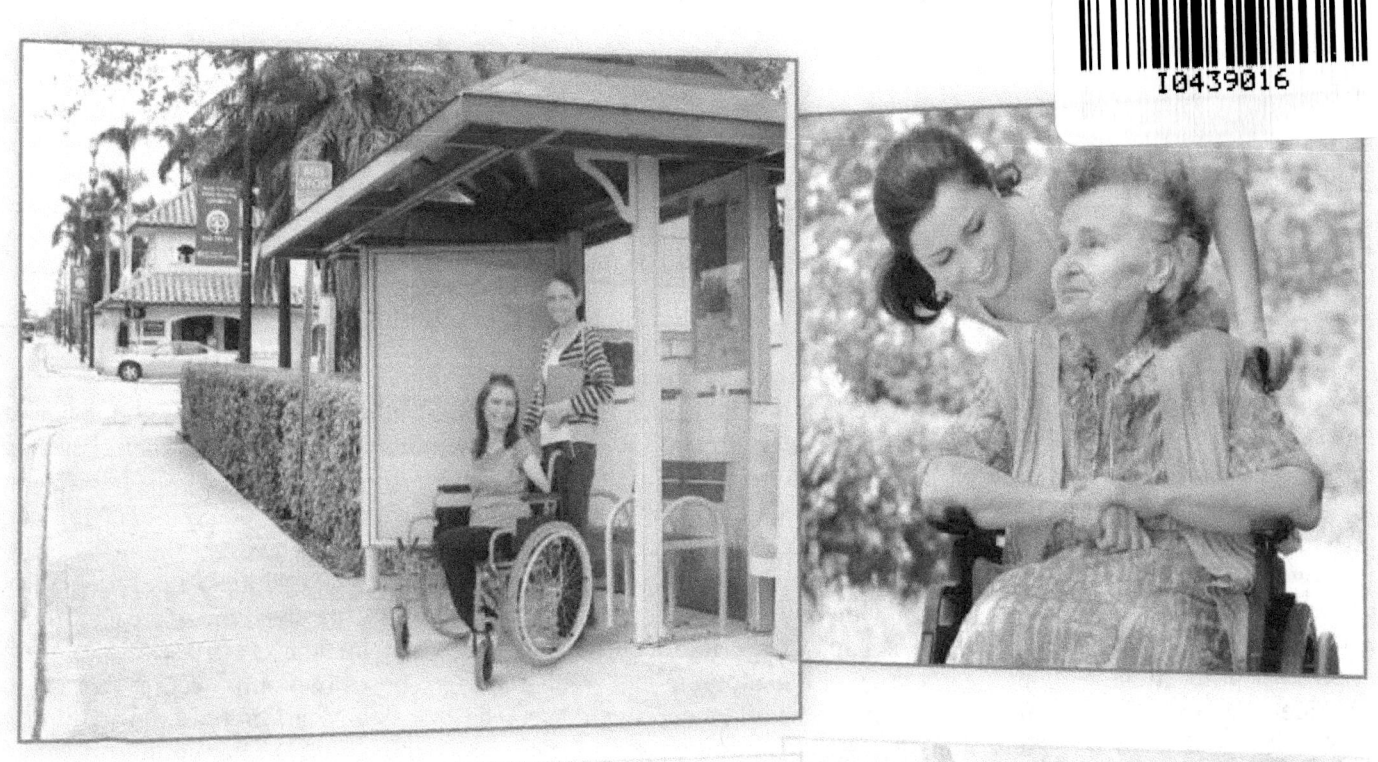

March 2010

http://www.fta.dot.gov/research

REPORT DOCUMENTATION PAGE

Form Approved
OMB No. 0704-0188

1. AGENCY USE ONLY (Leave blank)	2. REPORT DATE March 2010	3. REPORT TYPE AND DATES COVERED Final Report: July 2006-March 2010

4. TITLE AND SUBTITLE

Optimization Models for Prioritizing Bus Stop Facility Investments for Riders with Disabilities

5. FUNDING NUMBERS

6. AUTHOR(S)

Wanyang Wu, Albert Gan, Fabian Cevallos, and L. David Shen

7. PERFORMING ORGANIZATION NAME(S) AND ADDRESS(ES)

Lehman Center for Transportation Research
Florida International University
10555 W. Flagler Street, EC 3680, Miami, FL 33174

8. PERFORMING ORGANIZATION REPORT NUMBER

LCTR-TRANSPO-Year2-P2

9. SPONSORING/MONITORING AGENCY NAME(S) AND ADDRESS(ES)

Federal Transit Administration
U.S. Department of Transportation   Website: http://www.fta.dot.gov/research
Washington, DC 20590

10. SPONSORING/MONITORING AGENCY REPORT NUMBER

FTA-FL-04-7104-2010.03

11. SUPPLEMENTARY NOTES

Task Order Manager: Ms. Charlene Wilder
Federal Transit Administration
1200 New Jersey Avenue, SE, 4th Floor – East Building, E-43-420, Washington, DC 20590

12a. DISTRIBUTION/AVAILABILITY STATEMENT

In addition to FTA's method of distribution, this document will be made available though the Lehman Center for Transportation Research website at lctr.eng.fiu.edu

12b. DISTRIBUTION CODE

TRI-30

13. ABSTRACT (Maximum 200 words)

The Americans with Disabilities Act (ADA) of 1990 prescribes the minimum requirements for bus stop accessibility by riders with disabilities. Due to limited budgets, transit agencies can only select a limited number of bus stop locations for ADA improvements annually. These locations should preferably be selected such that they maximize the overall benefits to patrons with disabilities. In addition, transit agencies may choose to implement the "universal design" paradigm, which involves higher design standards than current ADA requirements and can provide amenities that are useful for all riders, like shelters and lighting. Many factors can affect the decision to improve a bus stop, including rider-based aspects like the number of riders with disabilities, total ridership, customer complaints, accidents, deployment costs, as well as spatial aspects like the location of employment centers, schools, shopping areas, and so on. These interlacing factors make it difficult to identify optimum improvement locations without the aid of an optimization model. This report proposes two optimization models to help identify a priority list of bus stops for accessibility improvements. The first is a binary integer programming model designed to identify bus stops that need improvements to meet the minimum ADA requirements. The second involves a multi-objective nonlinear mixed integer programming model that attempts to achieve an optimal compromise among the two accessibility design standards. Based on a case study using data from Broward County Transit (BCT) in Florida, the models were found to produce a list of bus stops that were determined to be highly logical upon close examination. Compared to traditional approaches using staff experience, requests from elected officials, customer complaints, etc., these optimization models offer a more objective and efficient platform on which to make bus stop improvement suggestions.

14. SUBJECT TERMS

Americans with Disabilities Act (ADA), Bus Stop Accessibility, Geographic Information Systems (GIS), Multi-Objective Optimization, Analytic Hierarchy Process

15. NUMBER OF PAGES

119

16. PRICE CODE

17. SECURITY CLASSIFICATION OF REPORT Unclassified	18. SECURITY CLASSIFICATION OF THIS PAGE Unclassified	19. SECURITY CLASSIFICATION OF ABSTRACT Unclassified	20. LIMITATION OF ABSTRACT

NSN 7540-01-280-5500
Prescribed by ANSI Std. 239-18298-102

Standard Form 298 (Rev. 2-89)

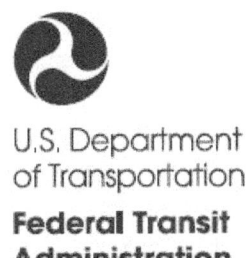

U.S. Department
of Transportation

**Federal Transit
Administration**

Optimization Models for Prioritizing Bus Stop Facility Investments for Riders with Disabilities

March 2010

Prepared by
Wanyang Wu, Albert Gan, Fabian Cevallos, and L. David Shen
Lehman Center for Transportation Research
Florida International University
10555 West Flagler Street, EC 3680
Miami, FL 33174
http://lctr.eng.fiu.edu/

Report No. **FTA-FL-04-7104-2010.03**

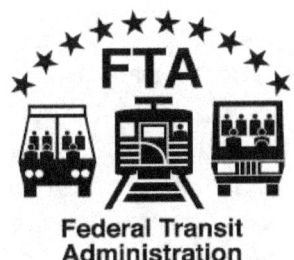

Federal Transit
Administration

Sponsored by
Federal Transit Administration
Office of Research, Demonstration, and Innovation
U.S. Department of Transportation
1200 New Jersey Avenue, SE
Washington, D.C. 20590

Available Online
[http://www.fta.dot.gov/research]

FOREWORD

This research was sponsored by the Federal Transit Administration (FTA) to develop a scientific method to help prioritize bus stops for accessibility improvements for riders with disabilities. To meet this objective, two optimization models were proposed and evaluated. Based on a case study using data from the Broward County Transit in Florida, the models were found to produce a list of bus stops that would extend the greatest benefits to riders with disabilities. This report details the process of identifying the bus stop accessibility requirements, identifying the factors affecting accessibility, preparing the required data for model input, formulating the optimization models, and evaluating the model performance. It is hoped that the proposed approach provides a more objective method of allocating the often limited resources for bus stop improvements.

DISCLAIMER NOTICE

ACKNOWLEDGEMENTS

The authors would like to acknowledge the financial support for this research from the Federal Transit Administration (FTA) of the United States Department of Transportation. The support was provided as part of the Center for Transportation Needs of Special Population (TRANSPO) Program of the Lehman Center for Transportation Research (LCTR) at Florida International University. The authors are grateful to their project manager, Ms. Charlene Wilder of the Federal Transit Administration (FTA), for her support and guidance throughout the project. Special thanks are due to Mr. Roberto Galvez and Ms. Adriana Toro of Broward County Transit (BCT), Florida for their advice and assistance in providing ridership and construction cost data used in this research; Dr. Jill Strube of the University of Texas at Austin for her review and editing of this report; and to Dr. Mary A. Leary and her staff members at Easter Seals Project ACTION for their review and thoughtful feedback.

TABLE OF CONTENTS

LIST OF FIGURES

LIST OF TABLES

EXECUTIVE SUMMARY

Introduction

Inaccessible bus stops prevent people with disabilities from using fixed-route bus services, thus limiting their mobility. Accessible design focuses on compliance with laws and regulations as well as state or local building codes. The law and regulations are intended to eliminate certain physical barriers that limit the usability of the built environment for people with disabilities. The Americans with Disabilities Act (ADA) of 1990 prescribes the minimum requirements for bus stop accessibility by riders with disabilities.

While ADA standards provide the minimum requirements in compliance with law, they are not necessarily "best practices." Easter Seals Project ACTION initiated the "universal design" concept for bus stops. The goal of universal design is to create environments that facilitate bus access, safety, and comfort for all transit users. Universal design provides a higher level of access for people with disabilities because, while consideration is given to people with disabilities under the minimum ADA standards, these considerations are not sufficient when planning and designing for the whole population. Universal design also benefits other people with reduced mobility, such as children, older adults, parents pushing strollers, people with temporary injuries, pregnant women, and even travelers pulling luggage. Universal design is a better choice than ADA minimum requirements if the public transit planning or improvement project has the requisite budget.

Although the accessibility improvements mandated under the ADA have enforceable regulations and standards, many bus stops still do not meet the mandate. One way for transit agencies to improve accessibility to transit systems for patrons with disabilities is to add to all bus stops ADA-compliant features such as curb cuts, sidewalks, loading pads, etc., as well as auditory messages such as talking signs and voice announcements. However, due to budget restrictions, transit agencies can only select a limited number of improvements at select bus stop locations for ADA improvements annually. In practice, locations for improvements are usually selected based on existing information, staff experience, and requests from elected officials. However, it is very difficult to identify locations that will benefit most from improvements amid considerations of funding, transit patronage, and existing facilities.

Many factors can affect the decision to improve a bus stop. These factors interlace and create optimum investment decisions that cannot be made using ordinary approaches. A decision-making tool that considers the effects of these factors is needed to maximize the benefits of bus stop improvements to riders with disabilities. Accordingly, this research study was aimed at developing optimization models that can better identify the types of improvements needed and determine the most effective locations for these improvements under budget constraints. Specifically, two optimization models were developed, one to meet only the minimum ADA requirements and another to achieve an optimal compromise among the minimum ADA and universal design standards.

Literature Review

A comprehensive literature search and review were performed to investigate and assess advances in state-of-the-art optimization models and various kinds of bus stop design standards and requirements. The purposes were: 1) to identify the problems facing riders with disabilities regarding bus stop accessibility; and 2) to determine evaluation criteria and optimization methods that will form the final research framework and tasks.

The Americans with Disabilities Act (ADA) of 1990 provided guidelines and minimum requirements regarding bus stop accessibility for persons with disabilities. Transit agencies must adhere to these requirements during new construction and improvements to existing facilities. The major concern of the ADA minimum requirements is to ensure that a given bus stop can provide adequate connections to the bus stop, as well as to enable boarding and disembarking for riders with disabilities. ADA minimum requirements focused on satisfying specific minimum technical criteria to allow most people with disabilities to use the built environment. By contrast, universal design concepts intend to provide a more comfortable environment than strict ADA adherence, including features like benches, shelters, lighting, etc., that additionally make the experience better for all transit users.

Most bus stop accessibility research has focused on bus stop location optimization, which is different from the focus on fixed-route bus stops in this research. However, some ideas presented in previous research are useful for the purposes of this study. One example is the location set covering problem (LSCP) model, which seeks to minimize the number of stops in one analysis region within which there will be at least one transit stop. Another example is the maximal covering location problem (MCLP) model that is used to maximize bus stop coverage from the standpoint of location. Also valuable to this research is the Los Angeles study which investigated and summarized the relationship between ridership, wait time, and the distribution of bus stop shelters. Likewise, the research on bus transit accessibility for people with reduced mobility provides a detailed list of measurable variables that can be treated as a reliable reference.

As a major potential approach for this study, spatial multicriteria decision making and its applications in transportation problems were fully reviewed. The entire framework and methodology, its objectives, and evaluation systems were found to be suitable for this research. Spatial analysis and the ActiveX interface of ArcGIS were introduced as they relate to the programming of optimization models.

Methodology

The methodology applied in this research consists of three main stages. During the first stage of development, a bus stop accessibility checklist based on ADA minimum requirements is used to evaluate existing bus stops. Bus stops, transit ridership, and socioeconomic data from three main data sources were collected and processed to generate evaluation criteria and alternatives. During the second stage, the analytical hierarchy process (AHP) was used to compare and evaluate different criteria and assign weights to bus stops. In the final stage, two optimization models using mathematical programming techniques were formulated to find the optimal total bus stop weights (combined with those from all criteria considered) that maximize the overall system benefit within a limited budget. The models were formulated such that all selected bus stops can be brought into compliance with minimum ADA accessibility standards as well. Major constraints were determined based on the budget allocations for bus stop accessibility improvement and construction costs for bus stop facilities.

Data Preparation

Broward County Transit (BCT) provided a bus stop status inventory that includes data on 5,034 bus stops. Using this inventory, a full checklist was developed to evaluate current bus stop conditions for riders with disabilities based on both the ADA minimum requirements and universal design standards. Ridership data, comprised of wheelchair boardings, general ridership based on bus stop location, and work trips by persons with disabilities, were included. Socioeconomic factors, including population statistics regarding persons with disabilities, as well as likely destinations and facilities were considered. The bus stop service area component was developed to integrate all the criteria. Factors that are interpreted as points were treated using a special arithmetic to solve the issue regarding closest distance in overlapping service areas. Correlation analysis was performed to identify the factors that were highly correlated. A user-friendly program was developed to perform all the calculations involved in AHP, making it easy for decision makers or planners to assign priority weights based on their judgment and experience.

A full cost estimation list for each candidate bus stop was established based on the ADA improvement budget of Broward County and the construction cost estimates for candidate bus stops based on estimates from current contractors. On this list, each bus stop has two different cost estimates based on both the minimum ADA and universal design standards. Besides the general cost for survey, labor organization, and maintenance of traffic, the cost of bus stop improvements for the minimum ADA standard includes that for sidewalks, loading pads, and curb cuts. The cost of bus stop improvements for universal design includes that for benches, lightings, shelters, bus maps, and schedules. The final list of the candidate bus stops also included 84 bus stop groups. These bus stop groups were developed to avoid duplication of calculation for sidewalk length and curb-cut because of shared sidewalks by multiple stops.

Optimization Models Development

Two different optimization models were developed for ADA bus stop improvements to meet two different objectives: 1) satisfying the minimum ADA standard, and 2) satisfying both objectives, i.e., the minimum ADA standards and the higher universal design standards. The former is a relatively simple binary linear programming model, and the latter mainly applies nonlinear mixed integer model in goal programming via the General Algebraic Modeling System (GAMS).

In the two optimization models, the corresponding relationship dataset between a candidate bus stop and a bus stop group was introduced to prevent duplication in cost calculation for sidewalk and curb-cut construction. The models assume that the selected bus stops will be made to fully meet the ADA accessibility requirements or the universal design requirements. Single improvements, such as building only a loading pad or a bench, are not allowed in each objective.

From the model output based on the BCT data, about 600 bus stops were selected for ADA improvement for the next funding cycle. The results show that a large percentage of the selected bus stops needed only minor investments to substantially benefit riders with disabilities. Because the model is a nonlinear mixed integer programming, it cannot ensure that every combination has a feasible solution. The single objective model is preferred if only the minimum ADA standards need to be met.

These two optimization models have different applicability. Based on the Broward County bus stop accessibility inventory, nearly half of the bus stops did not meet minimum ADA requirements with some needing only a minor investment to comply with ADA standards. Meeting the minimum ADA requirements should be the priority (rather than making the investment to meet the universal design standard) due to the limited County budget. Therefore, the single objective model that aims to meet the minimum ADA standard was more suitable for Broward County. On the other hand, if a large number of the bus stops for a transit agency were qualified under the minimum ADA standard, that agency might be able to improve the accessibility of a bus stop at the higher service level standard. The second model that aims to satisfy two objectives would be a better choice.

Sensitivity Analysis

The sensitivity analysis performed in this research shows that the optimization models are reasonable. The budget sensitivity analysis describes how the model is more efficient when the budget is lower because the model selected as many bus stops as possible with higher scores at lower cost. When the budget is higher, the benefit-cost ratios of the remaining candidate bus stops should be lower so the efficiency of the model will be lower. It also explains why over 600 bus stops were selected for improvement in the upcoming budget year. As BCT makes progress improving bus stops to meet ADA standards, the number of selected bus stops will decrease each year.

Factor sensitivity analysis was utilized to inspect how the changes in the weights for each factor will affect the optimization model. The model output shows that there were no breaking points for the factors. In other words, every weighted curve changed smoothly. When the ratio of each factor increased by 0.1, the model selected bus stops changed by 10 to 35 bus stops, while the total score basically remained constant. Compared to the other factors, religious centers, health centers, and schools caused larger changes to the optimization model.

Conclusions

In this research, a GIS-based decision support system was developed to allocate bus stop facility improvements for riders with disabilities. Using Broward County Transit data, a full bus stop accessibility checklist for riders with disabilities was developed based on an analysis of the ADA minimum requirements and universal design standards. By evaluating eight different criteria within every candidate bus stop service area, the analytical hierarchy process (AHP) calculated a single scenario with one simple number. Next, two different optimization models were developed for ADA bus stop improvements. One considered satisfying only the minimum ADA standards, while the other took into account two objectives—the minimum ADA standards and the higher standard of universal design. Based on the model output, about 600 bus stops would require ADA improvements during the next budget year.

These two optimization models have different applicability. Based on the Broward County bus stop accessibility inventory, nearly half of the bus stops did not meet minimum ADA requirements, with many needing only a minor investment to be ADA-compliant. Due to the limited County budget, meeting the minimum ADA requirements should take precedence over the higher investment needed by universal design. Therefore, the single objective model that aims to meet the minimum ADA standard was more suitable for Broward County. On the other hand, if a large number of the bus stops for a transit agency qualified under the minimum ADA standard, that agency might be able to improve the accessibility of bus stops at the higher service level standard. For these agencies, the second model that aims to satisfy two objectives would thusly be a better choice.

The two aspects of sensitivity analysis performed in this research, both budget and factor, show that the optimization models are reasonable. The budget sensitivity analysis illustrated how the model was more efficient when the budget was lower, while the factor sensitivity analysis was used to inspect how changes in the weight value affected the optimization model as a whole. Compared to the traditional approaches for bus stop selection which rely on staff experience, requests from elected officials, and customer complaints, these optimization models offer a decidedly more objective and efficient platform for bus stop improvement suggestions.

Recommendations

The following recommendations are made to further improve the results from the two optimization models developed in this research:

1. Make use of data with smaller spatial units, such as at the parcel level rather than at the census blockgroup or Traffic Analysis Zone (TAZs) level, in order to obtain more precise distance calculation between a trip origin (or destination) and the nearest bus stop.

2. Calibrate the intercept and slope parameters for the distance decay model to reflect those of the populations with disabilities, rather than those of the general population.

3. Allow multiple funding sources for each bus stop improvement type. For example, shelter and bench improvements may be funded by both ADA budget and advertisements.

4. Make use of additional variables, such as location and presence of obstacles, connection with other sidewalk, construction work hours needed, etc., in order to better estimate the sidewalk distance and their corresponding construction cost.

5. Expand the optimization models to consider improvements based on route, rather than on a single bus stop or a group of bus stops.

CHAPTER 1

INTRODUCTION

1.1. Background

The 2000 Census indicates that about 20 percent of the total population in the United States has some form of disability. Due to physical, sensory, or mental challenges, people with disabilities often depend on public transit as their primary source of transportation. However, inaccessible bus stops, which could be a result of poor design, physical barriers, topographical conditions, or lack of a sidewalk infrastructure, prevent riders with disabilities from using fixed-route bus services. Inaccessibility affects the mobility of riders with disabilities, lowers the efficiency of public transit, and increases the costs of other special transit services such as paratransit (Easter Seals Project ACTION, 2005).

Improving bus stop accessibility not only benefits riders with disabilities, but also enhances the usability of transit systems for all riders. For example, a comfortable shelter and bench can provide a rest area and protect passengers from bad weather; adequate lighting, furthermore, alleviates the security issues of using the bus at night, just as timely and accurate information reduces the ambiguity of the system. From a broader perspective, accessibility improvements should also be treated as affecting the general system usability. However, the National Council on Disability, a federal agency that advises the President and Congress, concluded that persistent problems still face people with disabilities who use public transportation despite years of federal efforts to make buses and trains more accessible (2004). The Easter Seals Project ACTION (2005) found that people with disabilities who need to use public transit systems are not being well served, despite billions of dollars spent to improve transportation for this demographic. Regarding bus stop accessibility, the report cited the following main problems:

- Wheelchair users face significant difficulties in moving and overcoming steps or pavement/platforms, as well as being forced to move on irregular, uneven surfaces;
- People with sensorial disabilities (sight, hearing, or speaking) have serious difficulties using conventional transport services (for example, getting to the bus stop, as well as boarding and alighting from the vehicle); and
- Some private bus shelter providers and the local governments that sign contracts with them may have no financial incentive (e.g., revenue from advertising) for locating bus shelters where the bus riders are—in the poorer, more transit-dependent areas of a city.

Figure 1-1 shows two bus stops: one is not accessible to patrons on wheelchairs while the other is considered fully accessible. Accessible design focuses on compliance with laws and regulations as well as state or local building codes. The laws and regulations are intended to eliminate certain physical barriers that limit the usability of the built environment for people with disabilities. In the past, these were typically based on requirements detailed by the American National Standards Institute. With the Americans with Disabilities Act (ADA) of 1990 and the subsequent ADA Accessibility Guidelines, accessible design has focused more on satisfying these minimum technical criteria to allow most people with disabilities to use the built environment.

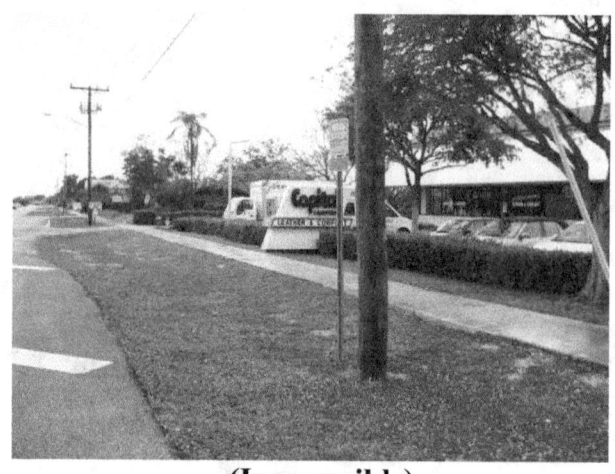 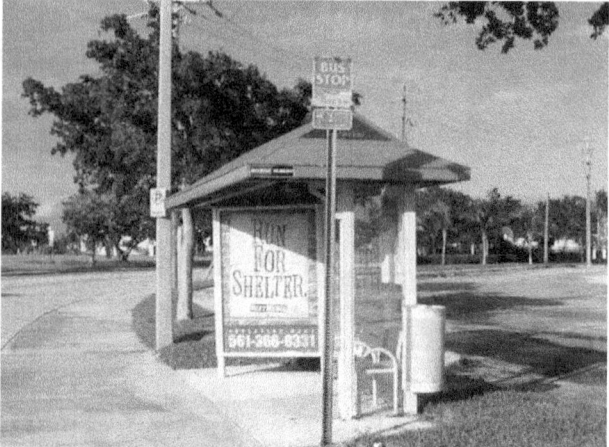

(Inaccessible) **(Fully Accessible)**

Figure 1-1 Examples Showing Inaccessible and Fully Accessible Bus Stops.

The ADA is broad legislation intended to make American society more accessible to people with disabilities (Department of Justice, 1994). It consists of five titles: employment, public services, public accommodations, telecommunications, and miscellaneous. Among these titles, Titles II and III (public services and public accommodations) affect bus stop planning, design, and construction. They focus on accessible paths, shelter, lighting, sign, and schedule information improvements that satisfy minimum technical criteria and allow most people with disabilities to use the bus stop environment.

While the ADA standards describe the minimum criteria required to comply with the law, they are not necessarily "best practices." The Easter Seals Project ACTION (2005) initiated the "universal design" concept for bus stops. The goal of universal design is to create environments suitable for all transit users. Universal design provides a higher level of access for people with disabilities because, while it employs the ADA minimum requirements, these minimum standards are not sufficient when planning and designing for the needs of these special populations. For example, ADA requirements do not specify lighting standards in bus stop design, but people with visual impairments have great difficulty distinguishing bus stops or schedule information at night or in overcast weather. Universal design also benefits other people with reduced mobility, including children, older adults, parents pushing strollers, individuals with temporary injuries, pregnant women, and even travelers pulling luggage. Universal design is a better choice than ADA minimum standards if the public transit planning or improvement project has the requisite budget.

1.2. Problem Statement

Although the accessibility improvements mandated under the ADA have enforceable regulations and standards, many bus stops do not meet the mandate. The results from a bus stop survey, for example, show that more than 15 years after the ADA was enacted, about a quarter of the bus stops in Palm Beach County, Florida still did not meet the minimum ADA requirements (LCTR, 2007). Clearly, one way for transit agencies to improve accessibility to transit systems for patrons with disabilities is to add to all bus stops ADA-compliant features such as curb-cuts, sidewalks, loading pads, etc., as well as auditory messages such as talking signs and voice announcements. However, agencies often have limited budgets and do not have the resources to improve accessibility at all bus stops. As such, these facilities should be installed in locations where patrons with disabilities will realize maximum benefits. In practice, locations for improvements are usually selected based on existing information, staff experience, and requests from elected officials. However, it is very difficult to identify locations that will benefit most from improvements under the constraints of available funds, transit patronage, and existing facilities.

Many factors can affect the decision to improve a bus stop, including rider-based aspects like total ridership, customer complaints, accidents, deployment costs, as well as spatial aspects like the location of employment centers, schools, shopping areas, and so on. These factors interlace and create optimum investment decisions that cannot be made using ordinary approaches. A decision-making tool that considers the effects of these factors is needed to more accurately identify the type of improvements required and to determine the most appropriate locations for the improvements.

1.3. Research Objective

The objective of this research is to develop a decision-making tool that can help identify the types of bus stop accessibility improvements needed and to determine the most effective locations for these improvements under budget constraints. This will be done by developing optimization models with the aid of a Geographic Information System (GIS). Specifically, two optimization models will be developed. The first model aims to meet only the minimum ADA requirements, while the second model aims to achieve an optimal compromise among the minimum ADA and universal design standards. Both models make use of information in existing transit databases (including bus stop inventory, transit ridership, wheelchair ridership, customer complaints, accidents, etc.), facility deployment costs, service area demographic information, and land use parcel data for workplace locations.

1.4. Report Organization

This report consists of a total of seven chapters. Chapter 1 introduces the background of this research, describes the major problems to be solved, and sets the objective to be achieved.

Chapter 2 presents an extensive literature review covering the accessibility standards from ADA and university design for bus stops, public transit pattern study for people with disabilities, current research on spatial multicriteria decision making and the application software. The purpose of this review is to understand all regulations and standards on bus stop improvements for riders with disabilities, as well as the relative research and experience of other investigators on the subject.

Chapter 3 identifies the problems that need to be solved and determines two major objectives for the two optimization models to be developed. One is to meet the minimum ADA standards, and the other reaches for a higher standard—universal design. This chapter also discusses a feasible strategy to develop an optimization model, the major data sources, and the optimization method.

Chapter 4 explains the data collection and integration process. Ridership data and socioeconomic criteria are analyzed and integrated into a "bus stop status inventory." This chapter also introduces an analytic hierarchy process to combine the criteria considered and generates the overall score for evaluating the accessibility of each bus stop. Finally, through a case study, this chapter explains Broward County's ADA improvement budget and the construction cost estimates for candidate bus stops based on current contract information.

Chapter 5 describes the process of developing two different optimization models for bus stop improvements: one focuses on meeting the minimum ADA standards, the other seeks to compromise between the minimum ADA standards and the universal design.

Chapter 6 presents a comprehensive model sensitivity analysis on the budget changes and the different weight combinations for each factor considered in the models.

Finally, Chapter 7 summarizes the major research results in each chapter, draws conclusions, and recommends issues for future research.

CHAPTER 2

LITERATURE REVIEW

This chapter presents an extensive literature review covering ADA standards, the universal bus stop design concept and basic requirements, public transit pattern studies about riders with disabilities, and current research and software on spatial multicriteria decision-making procedures.

2.1. Checklists for Accessibility Requirements

The first step to determining and implementing bus stop improvements is to identify the conditions and facilities at and around bus stops. This can be done with a bus stop accessibility checklist. The checklists for meeting minimum ADA requirements and universal design standards are provided below.

2.1.1. Checklists for Minimum ADA Requirements for Bus Stop Amenities

The Americans with Disabilities Act (ADA) of 1990 outlines the minimum requirements that persons with disabilities require at bus stops. As such, it is the most important design reference for transit stop inventory. Title II of the ADA covers sidewalk and street construction and transit accessibility, referencing the ADA Accessibility Guidelines (ADAAG) or the Uniform Federal Accessibility Standards (UFAS) for new construction and alterations undertaken by or on behalf of a state or local government (Federal Transit Administration, 1992). In addition, the Department of Justice (1994) Title II regulation specifically requires that curb ramps be provided when sidewalks or streets are newly constructed or altered. Details regarding these requirements are listed below.

Bus Stop Area and Bus Landing Pads

A bus stop platform is a designated bus stop area clear of obstructions to facilitate boarding and disembarking for all users. It must meet the following criteria:

- The platform must be a firm, stable surface.
- It must have a minimum clear length of 96 inches (2,440 millimeters), measured from the curb or vehicle roadway edge, and a clear width of at least 60 inches (1,524 millimeters), measured parallel to the roadway.
- The platform may only have a maximum slope of 1:50 (2 percent) perpendicular to the roadway for water drainage.
- The platform pad must be connected to streets, sidewalks, or pedestrian paths by an accessible route.

Bus Shelter

New bus shelters must be installed or older ones replaced to accommodate wheelchair or mobility aided users, as follows:

- The bus shelter must have a minimum clear floor area of 30 by 48 inches (762 by 1,219 millimeters), entirely within the perimeter of the shelter.
- An accessible route to the boarding area or landing pad must connect it.

Additionally,

- Bus stop shelters should not be placed on the wheelchair landing pad.
- General ADA mobility clearance guidelines should be followed around the shelter and between the shelter and other street fixtures.
- A clearance of 36 inches (914 millimeters) should be maintained around the shelter and an adjacent sidewalk (more is preferred).
- Advertising panels should be located downstream of the traffic flow to allow an approaching bus driver to view the interior of the shelter easily. Indirect surveillance from passing traffic should be preserved through proper placement of the panels.

Lighting and Security

There are no specific ADA requirements for lighting and security.

Accessible Path

At minimum, an accessible path should fulfill the following criteria:

- It should have a minimum clear passage width of 48 inches (1,219 millimeters), as recommended by the Access Board's guidelines for the public right-of-way. This is especially important next to a curb drop-off.
- There should be an accessible link route from public transportation stops to the route for the general public.
- The maximum cross slope should be 1:50.
- The ground and floor surfaces should be stable, firm, and slip-resistant.
- Grating spaces should be no greater than 1/2 inch (13 millimeters) wide in one direction.

Objects may not protrude on an accessible route or maneuvering space. Guidelines for protruding objects are stated below:

- Objects projecting from walls (for example, telephones) with their leading edges between 27 inches and 80 inches (685 millimeters and 2,030 millimeters) above the finished floor shall protrude no more than 4 inches (100 millimeters) into the pathway.
- Objects mounted with their leading edges at or below 27 inches (685 millimeters) above the finished floor may protrude any amount.
- Free-standing objects mounted on posts or pylons may overhang 12 inches (305 millimeters) maximum from 27 inches to 80 inches (685 millimeters to 2,030 millimeters) above the ground or finished floor.

- Clear headroom should be 80 inches (2,030 millimeters) at minimum. If vertical clearance of an area adjoining an accessible route is less than 80 inches (nominal dimension), a barrier should be provided to warn blind or visually-impaired persons.

Route and Timetable Information, Transit Signage

Bus stop signage should fulfill the following criteria:

- Letters and numbers should have a width-to-height ratio between 3:5 and 1:1 and a stroke-width-to-height ratio between 1:5 and 1:10.
- Characters and numbers should be sized according to the viewing distance from which they are to be read.
- The minimum letter height is measured using an upper case X. Lower case characters are permitted.
- Signs should have accompanying pictograms with the equivalent verbal description placed directly below. A border dimension of 6 inches (152 millimeters) at minimum height should be around the signs.
- Characters and sign backgrounds should have a non-glare finish, with characters and symbols contrasting from their background.
- Signage should follow protruding objects requirements as discussed in the Accessible Path section.

Amenities

If benches are provided, they should adhere to the following ADA regulations:

- Clear floor or ground space for wheelchairs (complying with ADAAG Section 4.2.4).
- Seat dimensions: 20 inches (510 millimeters) minimum to 24 inches (610 millimeters) maximum in depth and 42 inches (1,065 millimeters) minimum in length.
- Seat height: 17 inches (430 millimeters) minimum to 19 inches (485 millimeters) maximum above the floor or ground.
- Back support: 42 inches (1,065 mm) minimum in length extending from a point 2 inches (51 mm) maximum above the seat to a point 18 inches (455 mm) minimum above the seat.
- Structure supporting vertical or horizontal forces of 250 pounds (1,112 Newtons) applied at any point on the seat, fastener, mounting device, or supporting structure.
- Exposed benches must be slip resistant and designed to shed water.

Also note that vending machines, newspaper boxes, trash receptacles, and other street fixtures must not reduce the minimum ADA requirements.

Communications

While including public telephones is not required, if they are provided, they must adhere to the following criteria:

- Persons using wheelchairs should be able to access at least one telephone. It must be located so that the receiver, coin slot, and control are no more than 48 inches (1,219 millimeters) above the floor.
- Clear floor or ground space must be at least 30 inches by 48 inches (762 millimeters by 1,219 millimeters), not impeded by bases, enclosures, or fixed seats, and must allow either a forward or parallel approach by a person using a wheelchair.
- The highest operable part of the telephone and telephone books should be within the reach ranges specified in ADAAG Sections 4.2.5 or 4.2.6.
- Locations must follow guidelines detailed in the section on Accessible Paths.
- Phones must be hearing aid compatible and volume control equipped in accordance with ADAAG Section 4.1.3.
- The cord must be a minimum of 29 inches (735 millimeters) long.

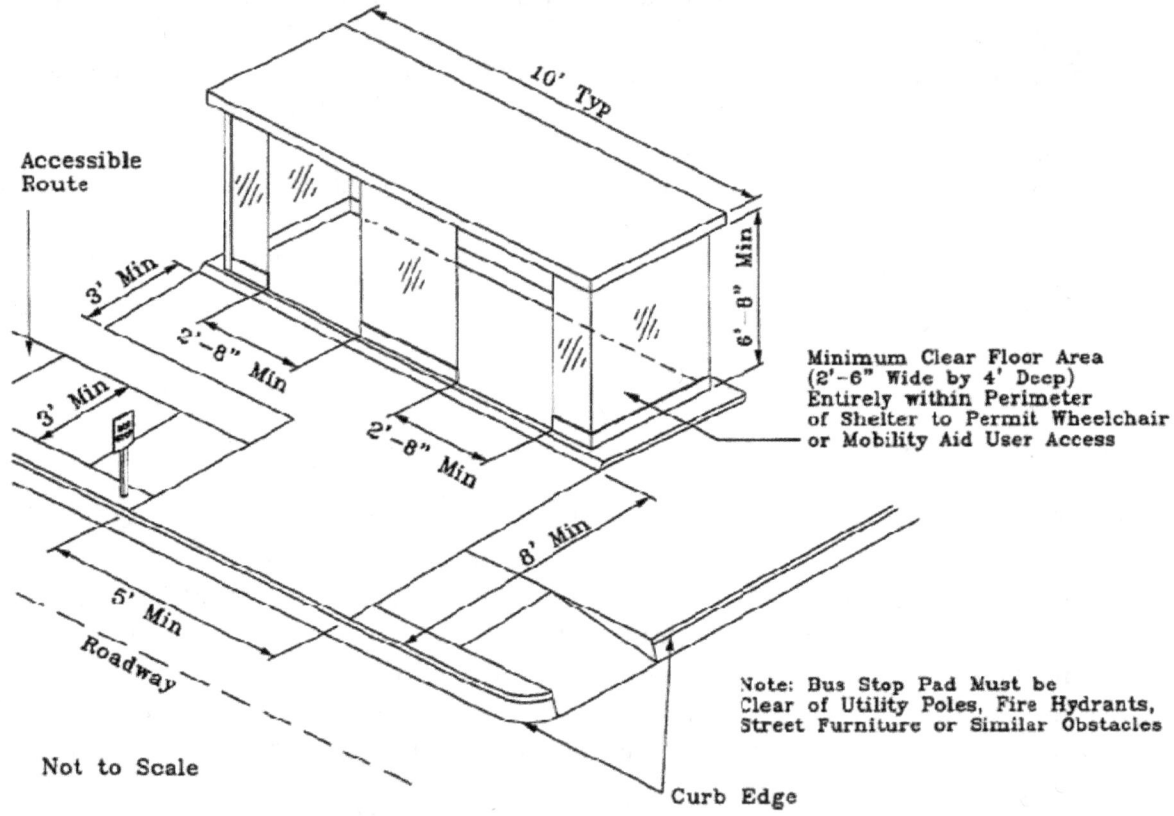

Figure 2-1 Example of a Bus Stop Design Example that Meets ADA Requirements (TCRP Report 19, 1996).

Identification of a Bus Stop by People with Visual Impairments

Although no specific ADA regulations require that people with visual disabilities be able to distinguish a bus stop from other street facilities, unique features should be added and incorporated into the design of each bus stop. Stops that have shelters are more readily identifiable due to the unique features of the shelter. However, bus stops only identifiable with signs on a utility pole can be difficult to discern. To address this issue, all locations should utilize a pole design unique to bus stops. For example, the pole may be square with holes running down its length. Where a unique pole is provided, the transit agency can educate customers who have visual impairments about this feature.

2.1.2. Checklists for Universal Design Standards for Bus Stop Amenities

As mentioned in Chapter 1, the Easter Seals Project ACTION initiated the "universal design" concept in 2005 to create built environments more suitable for all transit users. The ADA bus shelter standards provide a good example of the universal design concept. Minimum ADA requirements only mention that new bus shelters must be installed or older ones replaced to accommodate riders using wheelchairs or mobility aids. The requirements do not specify when agencies should install a shelter for a bus stop. Unlike the loading pad and the sidewalk width requirements, bus shelters are not necessary to meet minimum ADA standards. Universal design suggests that shelters be installed based on minimum boardings given in Table 2-1. Shelter design is based on criteria related to climate, agency size, community policies, and streetscape context. The following are general design guidelines that assist in providing accessibility and safety:

- Build shelters 9 feet long by 5 feet wide (2.7 meters by 1.5 meters).
- Design shelters with transparent sides for visibility and security.
- Mark glass panels with distinctive patterns such as horizontal contrasting strips or circles, to indicate the presence of the panels.
- Include transit route maps, schedules, and seating in shelters. People in wheelchairs and, to the greatest extent possible, persons with visual impairments should be able to read maps and schedules easily.
- Provide seating, if feasible, with sufficient space to move around.
- Provide surfaces to lean against if seating is not provided.
- Omit steps between the sidewalk/bus pad and the shelter.
- Maintain shelter openings at 36 inches (914 millimeters) minimum to allow a wheelchair to pass through.
- Consider heated shelters at high ridership stops in cold climates.

Table 2-1 Recommended Minimum Boardings to Install Shelter.

Location	Minimum boardings
Rural	10 boardings per day
Suburban	25 boardings per day
Urban	50 to 100 boardings per day

Lighting and Security

While bus riders with visual impairments benefit when bus stops have good lighting, proper lighting increases the safety and security of the stop to the benefit of all users (**Easter Seals Project ACTION**, 2005). The specific design guidelines include:

- Installing lighting that provides between 2 to 5 footcandles. A footcandle is a unit of luminance on a surface that is a uniform point source of light of one candela and equal to one lumen per square foot.
- Multiple sources of light are provided to avoid direct shadows. Lighting that is too bright in bus shelters can also compromise personal safety, creating a fish bowl effect whereby the transit user can easily be seen by others but cannot see outside.
- Avoid using exposed bulbs or similar lighting equipment that can be easily tampered with or destroyed, and ensure light facilities are easy to maintain.
- Bus stops are best located near existing streetlights for indirect lighting.

Passenger security is a major issue in bus stop design and location choice (TCRP Report 19, 1996), because it can positively or negatively influence passengers' perception of the bus stop. From a security point of view, bus stop facilities should avoid restricted sight lines. The specific design guidelines include:

- Construction materials for bus shelters should provide clear, unobstructed visibility to passengers waiting inside.
- Bus stops should be located at highly visible sites to allow approaching bus drivers and passing vehicles to clearly see the bus stop. Locations near stores and businesses also enhance surveillance of the site.
- For landscaping, elements without visual barriers are preferred at bus stops; for example, low-growing shrubbery, ground cover, and deciduous shade trees are best for these purposes.
- Bus stops should be coordinated with existing street lighting to improve visibility.
- Public works crews should remove obstacles that affect visibility and maintain the cleanliness of the bus stop.
- Bus stops should provide a pay phone or police call box for emergency calls.
- Bus stops should provide detailed bus route and schedule information.

Accessible Paths

Compared the guidelines required to meet the minimum ADA standards, universal design requirements are more stringent, especially regarding the width of sidewalk, the surfacing materials considered less difficult for the persons with visual impairments, and grade-level changes (Alberta Transportation Ministry, 2001). The specific design guidelines for accessible paths include:

- The width of sidewalk should be five or more feet to accommodate pedestrian or wheelchair users' activity in two directions.
- Public works crews should maintain walkways and bus stop areas, clearing them of trash, brush, snow, ice, and other debris.
- An accessible travel path should be provided from the bus stop to the sidewalk or accessible buildings.
- Guidelines specify special surface layer materials that persons with visual impairments can distinguish. These textures include: concrete, paving stones, contrasting colors, tactile strips, and curbs to help delineate pathways.

- On-street conveniences, such as benches, sign posts, and newspaper boxes, should be off the travel path of transit passengers.
- Pathway junction points should be defined and clear of obstructions.
- Curb ramps should be provided on any locations with grade-level changes because grade-level changes are difficult for older adults and persons with disabilities to negotiate.

Route, Timetable Information and Transit Signage

Universal design emphasizes the easy identification and durability of route, timetable information, and transit signage (TCRP Report 19, 1996). Recommendations for signage and route information displays are as follows:

- Update when changes are made to routes and schedules.
- Make permanent route and timetable information displays.
- Design shelters and stops to accommodate route and schedule information to avoid reduced visibility or security.
- Place route and timetable information on shelter interior side panels.
- Include backlighting for nighttime display.
- Provide real-time information display boards at key stops to give passengers the information on bus arrival times and delays. For people with visual impairments, include a button for audio information.
- Provide double-sided signs that can be seen in both directions and illuminated signs for nighttime visibility.
- Locate bus stop signs where people board the front door of the bus. The bottom of the sign should be at least 7 feet (2.1 meters) above ground level and should not be located closer than 2 feet (0.6 meters) from the curb face.
- Do not obstruct bus signs with trees, buildings, or other signs.

Amenities

Besides the dimension requirements for minimum ADA standards, universal design considers bench safety, comfort, and location. The following recommendations coordinate bench placement with the bus stop environment to enhance safety and accessibility (TCRP Report 19, 1996):

- Provide 17-inch (430 millimeter) high benches. Higher benches will be uncomfortable for many passengers.
- Locate benches under shady trees if possible. Otherwise, landscaping should protect passengers from the wind and other elements. Uncomfortable bus stop environmental conditions, such as heat or sun, can discourage bench use.
- Coordinate bench locations with existing streetlights to increase visibility and enhance security at the stop.
- Provide grab handles along the bench for older adult users or passengers with disabilities to use as support when standing up.
- Locate benches away from driveways to enhance safety and comfort.

- Maintain a minimum separation of 24 inches (610 millimeters) between the bench and the back-face of the curb. As the traffic speed of the adjacent road increases, increase the distance from the bench to the curb to ensure patron safety and comfort.
- Do not locate benches on wheelchair landing pads.
- Avoid metal seating surfaces. Those surfaces are very cold in winter and very hot in summer.

Communications

Universal design guidelines recognize that telephones at bus stops also create opportunities for illegal or unintended activities, such as drug dealing and loitering, which compromise passenger safety around bus stops. Recommended guidelines for placing telephones at bus stops include the following (TCRP Report 19, 1996):

- Separate the phone and the bus stop waiting area by a short distance if possible.
- Remove the return phone number attached to the phone.
- Limit the phone to outbound calls only.

2.2. Research on the Public Transit Pattern for Persons with Disabilities

Several studies have been undertaken to examine the travel patterns of people with disabilities who use public transit to establish which bus stops are near common destinations (such as hospitals, schools, and churches). These bus stops should get priority for ADA accessibility improvements.

The Scottish Executive Transport Research Planning Group (2006) commissioned research to support their commitment to assessing public transport options for persons with disabilities and to better target funding. Originally, the report focused on the role of concessionary fares in relation to the accessibility of transport for travelers with disabilities to inform the commitment described in the 2003 Scottish Executive Partnership Agreement. Advice from the Advisory Group broadened the scope at a very early stage. As a result, the research was changed to explore and assess a wide range of potential improvements to public transport for persons with disabilities. The researchers administered a face-to-face questionnaire survey of 700 Scottish residents who described themselves as having disabilities or a long-term illness. The sample for the project specific survey included people with a broad range of travel patterns and experiences. Table 2-2 shows the frequency of certain journey types. The results indicate that what might be deemed 'essential journeys,' such as shopping or visiting a doctor, are much more common than social visits. A considerable proportion of people with disabilities never travel for evening leisure purposes (64 percent), daytime leisure purposes (60 percent), or travel on holidays or for weekend getaways (around 50 percent each). Visiting friends or relatives is more common, suggesting that such journeys are shorter or easier (or are perhaps facilitated by friends or family).

Table 2-2 Different Journey Types (Frequency).

Base: All Respondents Undertaking At Least One Type of Journey At Least Occasionally	Most Days (%)	At Least Once a Week (%)	At Least Once a Month (%)	A Few Times a Year (%)	Less Often (%)	Never (%)
Day center or similar	1	6	2	< 5	1	90
Work/training or education	10	5	< 5	1	1	83
Evening leisure	2	15	9	7	4	64
Daytime leisure	9	20	5	3	4	60
Away for weekend	0	1	4	26	20	50
Away for holiday	0	0	0	13	37	49
Other medical visits	< 5	2	9	29	13	48
Convenience store/local shop	29	35	5	2	4	25
Personal business	2	48	23	5	3	20
Hospital appointments	< 5	2	9	43	29	17
Supermarket shopping	9	61	12	1	1	14
Visit friend or relatives	11	41	17	12	6	13
Visit Doctors	< 5	5	43	39	8	5

Source: TNS Survey 2005

The Bureau of Transportation Statistics (BTS), an operating administration within the U.S. Department of Transportation, set out to fill this data gap by developing and conducting the 2002 National Transportation Availability and Use Survey (2003). The purpose of this survey was to gather data and conduct research on identifying the transportation habits and needs of America's general population, establish a national dataset to allow analysis of the specific transportation habits and needs of people with disabilities, and provide contrasts with the population without disabilities. Faced with a wide spectrum of transportation demands, planners and policy makers need information to determine where transportation investments should be made. The survey was designed to identify the impact of transportation on the work and social lives of people with disabilities, and the extent to which it is unique to that population. The survey topics included:

- The number of people with disabilities who never leave their homes due to inadequate transportation alternatives;
- The types of transportation that people with disabilities use for local and long-distance travel;
- Their level of satisfaction with the system's ability to provide safe, accessible, reliable, efficient, and affordable transportation; and
- The barriers or challenges that the transportation environment, infrastructure, or vehicles pose.

All data presented in this survey were weighted to national totals. The data analysis summary compared two population groups—one comprised of people with disabilities and one comprised of people without disabilities. It also compared and contrasted challenges encountered by the two groups in their daily and non-routine travels and presented opinions regarding their transportation experiences. Table 2-3 shows the percent of types of trips that respondents with disabilities made via different types of transportation.

Table 2-3 Types of Trips Made by Respondents with Disabilites.

Type of Transportation	Work or Volunteer (%)	School (%)	Doctor and Medical Visits (%)	Other Local Travel (Shopping and Recreation) (%)
Personal motor vehicle as driver	66.37	26.99	53.11	52.44
Personal motor vehicle as passenger	15.18	21.07	36.84	36.43
Carpool or vanpool/group car/van	1.91	3.41	0.60	0.62
Public bus	5.34	3.68	3.36	3.35
Walking/nonmotorized wheelchair	2.93	5.98	1.37	2.77

Source: U.S. Department of Transportation, Bureau of Transportation Statistics, 2002 National Transportation Availability and Use Survey

The survey showed that people use multiple modes of transportation for local travel (Collia *et al.*, 2003). About 66 percent of people with disabilities who are 15 years or older, and about 86 percent of people who do not have disabilities and are 15 years or older, drove motor vehicles in the month prior to the interview for local travel—to work, to shop, to visit a physician , and for other purposes. Seventy-seven percent of those with disabilities and 82 percent of people without disabilities rode in a personal motor vehicle as a passenger for local travel. A greater proportion of persons without disabilities used carpools, vanpools, or group cars or vans (14 percent), school buses (11 percent), and subway, light rail, or commuter trains (9 percent) than persons with disabilities (11 percent, 5 percent, and 6 percent, respectively) for local travel.

Of the transportation typically provided to assist people with disabilities, only 6 percent used motorized personal transportation, such as electric wheelchairs, scooters or golf carts; 6 percent used paratransit vans or buses sponsored by the public transit authority; and 3 percent used specialized transportation services provided by human services agencies. However, driver status affected the type of transportation used. It was found that the proportion of respondents with and without disabilities who did not drive used carpools, taxicabs, and public transit more often than the proportion of respondents with and without disabilities who did drive.

With regard to trip purpose, although workers both with and without disabilities most often used personal motor vehicles to commute to paid or volunteer work, more workers with disabilities rode as passengers (15 percent) than did workers without disabilities (6 percent), while more individuals without disabilities drove (85 percent) than did individuals with disabilities (66 percent). Motor vehicles and school buses served as the primary transportation mode for commuting to school for both those with disabilities and those without. In addition, about one-quarter of both students with disabilities and without rode a school bus, and another quarter drove a motor vehicle to school most frequently. However, 36 percent of students without disabilities rode as a passenger in a personal motor vehicle compared to 21 percent of the students with disabilities.

Most individuals both with and without disabilities used motor vehicles, either as a driver or passenger, for transportation to the medical visits and for other local travel, such as shopping and recreation. About 2 to 3 percent of those with and without disabilities used a public bus for these trips. Although traveling by public transit represented only 2 to 5 percent of the total travel, the people with disabilities were found to use public transit at a much higher rate than the people without disabilities for each trip purpose.

On availability of public transportation, services were generally available to both those with disabilities and those without from their homes. For both groups, more than 50 percent lived near a sidewalk or path, almost 60 percent had public paratransit available in the area, and over three quarters had taxi service. About 25 percent lived within five miles of a subway, light rail, or commuter train station. Slightly more of the people with disabilities (47 percent) lived within one-quarter mile of a bus stop than did those without disabilities (42 percent).

The 2001 National Household Travel Survey (NHTS) is a good source for analyzing the travel patterns of older Americans. The main objective of this survey was to highlight travel patterns of older adults living in the United States as depicted in the 2001 NHTS. The NHTS is a national data collection program sponsored by the Bureau of Transportation Statistics and the Federal Highway Administration (FHWA). It was the first national comprehensive household survey of both daily and long-distance travel, allowing for the analysis of the full continuum of personal travel by Americans. To better understand the transportation needs of older Americans, it is useful to examine how travel patterns differ across age groups. The intent was to present basic travel characteristics of older adults (age 65+) and allow for comparisons with younger adults (ages 19-64). Both of these age groups were found to make many daily trips for family and personal reasons such as shopping, running errands, and recreational activities (see Table 2-4). Social and recreational trips, such as visiting friends, accounted for the largest percentage of older adults' trips (19 percent). Older adults took a significantly higher percentage of daily trips for shopping as compared to younger adults (18 percent and 13 percent respectively). Older adults also made a higher percentage of trips for medical reasons as compared to younger adults (3 percent and 1 percent respectively), and for religious reasons (3 percent and 1 percent respectively). As would be expected, work and work-related travel was found to constitute only a small percentage of daily travel for older adults as compared to their younger counterparts (3 percent versus 16 percent).

Table 2-4 Daily Travel: Distribution of Trips by Trip Purpose.

Purpose	Age: 19-64		Age: 65+	
	Percent	Standard Error	Percent	Standard Error
Work/work-related	16.1	0.15	3.1	0.19
Shopping	13.2	0.14	18.3	0.38
Family/personal business	16.4	0.15	17.5	0.29
School	0.9	0.04	0.1	0.04
Religious	1.3	0.04	2.6	0.13
Medical/dental	1.3	0.04	2.9	0.11
Social/recreation	17.1	0.15	19.4	0.30
Return home	32.7	0.10	34.8	0.25
Other	1.0	0.04	1.2	0.10
Total	100.0	-	100.0	-

Source: The 2001 National Household Travel Survey, Daily Trip File, U.S. Department of Transportation.

2.3. Bus Stop Facility Configurations in Different Areas

Bus stop facilities need not always be uniform. Some facilities are not necessary in rural or low-density areas. These include shelters, benches, lighting, vending machines, etc. Besides satisfying the ADA minimum requirements, different studies have shown that there were different local standards for bus stop facilities. Easter Seals Project ACTION (2005) divided bus stop shelter installations into three groups based on minimum boarding: rural (10 boardings per day), suburban (25 boardings per day), and urban (50-100 boardings per day). Law and Taylor (2001) used a point system to evaluate whether a bus stop shelter is necessary, dividing a system into six levels; the lowest level scored four points to indicate 0-50 daily boardings. The highest level indicated 400 or more daily boardings. A report by the Florida Planning and Development Lab (2004) determined that population and land use can establish standards for different kinds of bus stop facilities (see Table 2-5).

Table 2-5 Development Thresholds and Bus Stop Facilities.

Developer Thresholds	Required Facilities
Developments greater than 500,000 sq. ft. or 1,000 residential units	• Sidewalks • ADA and paratransit access • Sheltered Park-and-Ride facility • Separate bus loading and unloading area • Bus staging area for passenger loading/unloading
Developments of 500 to 1,000 residential units; Non-residential and mixed use developments of 200,000 - 500,000 sq. ft.	• Sidewalks • ADA and paratransit access • Bus bay • Transit accessory pad w/shelter, seating, trash receptacle, and bicycle rack
Non-residential developments 100,000 -200,000 sq. ft.	• Sidewalks • ADA and paratransit access • Transit accessory pad w/shelter, seating, trash receptacle, and bicycle rack
Non-residential developments 50,000 -100,000 sq. ft.	• Sidewalks • ADA and paratransit access • Transit accessory pad w/shelter, seating, trash receptacle, and bicycle rack
Non-residential developments or single- or multi-tenant office buildings of less than 50,000 sq. ft.	• Sidewalks • ADA and paratransit access • Pedestrian and bicycle connections

Other studies on bus stop accessibility in Europe are good references when developing bus stop inventories. One study in Oviedo, Spain ('Olio et al., 2007) aimed at bus transit accessibility for people with reduced mobility (broadening the concept of "reduced mobility" from only persons with disabilities to include children, older adults, and pregnant women). Table 2-6 shows all of the measured variables (including route variables) used in this study. To assess the accessibility problems in Oviedo's urban public transport system in greater detail, a questionnaire was developed to collect passengers' attitudes regarding the comfort and location of bus stops, access to stops and buses, drivers' attitudes, and vehicle equipment.

Table 2-6 Measured Variables and Route Variables.

Measured Variables	
Bus routes covered by the stop	Existence of a shelter
Type of shelter	State of the shelter
Comfort of the stop	Comfort in inclement weather
Notice board (yes/no)	Presence of pavement
Height of pavement	Width of pavement
Width of pavement in front of the stop	Width of pavement behind the stop
Length of slope of pavement	Width of slope of pavement
Isolated stop (yes/no)	Night use
Lighting	Presence of obstacles
Easy access for people with reduced mobility	Presence of parking bay
Maximum length of bay	Minimum length of parking bay
Width of bay	Entrance side of parking bay
Departure side of parking bay	Length of pull up for the bus (meters)
Type of pavement	State of pavement
Nearby pedestrian crossing	Presence of way out
Slope of way out	Lifting ramps
Route Variables	
Number of the bus route	Number of stops
Distance covered by the route	Average demand during rush hours
Average daily demand	Total of outgoing departures
Total of return departures	Average outgoing speed
Average return speed	Minimum outgoing time
Minimum return time	Average outgoing frequency
Average return frequency	

2.4. Transit Service Optimization and Relevant Issues

2.4.1. Optimization Models for Transit Service Accessibility Analysis

Various optimization models have been used to evaluate transit service accessibility. One model is the location set covering problem (LSCP) utilized by Murray (2003) and first proposed by Toregas *et al.* (1971). The objective function of LSCP is as follows:

$$Min \sum_i x_j \qquad (2\text{-}1)$$

subject to

$$\sum_{j \in N_i} x_j \geq 1 \quad \forall \ i \qquad (2\text{-}2)$$

$$x_j = (0,1) \quad \forall \ j \qquad (2\text{-}3)$$

where

i = the index of areas providing suitable access,

j = the index of transit stops,

$N_i = \{j \mid d_{ij} \leq S\}$, i.e., the number of transit stops in area i with d_{ij} shorter than S,

d_{ij} = the shortest distance between area i and stop j,

S = the service access distance standard, and

$$x_j = \begin{cases} 1 & \text{if an existing transit stop is to be included in system,} \\ 0 & \text{otherwise} \end{cases}$$

The objective of the LSCP is to minimize the number of stops needed in the bus transit system. Constraint (2-2) ensures that every service area along a route or in the analysis region will be provided at least one transit stop for suitable service. Constraint (2-3) is an integer restriction that determines whether a stop is kept in the system or removed.

Church and ReVelle (1974) proposed the maximal covering location problem (MCLP) to take ridership and operational costs into account. The formulation of the MCLP is as follows:

$$Max \sum_i a_i y_i \tag{2-4}$$

subject to

$$\sum_{j \in N_i} x_j \geq y_i \tag{2-5}$$

$$\sum_j x_j = p \tag{2-6}$$

$$x_j = (0,1) \quad \forall \ j \tag{2-7}$$

$$y_i = (0,1) \quad \forall \ i$$

where

a_i = current/anticipated ridership in area i,

p = the number of transit stops to select, and

$$y_j = \begin{cases} 1 & \text{if area } i \text{ has suitable access to a stop,} \\ 0 & \text{otherwise.} \end{cases}$$

The objective of the MCLP for public transit service analysis is to maximize the total proportion of a population (or public transit users) that will receive service coverage. Constraint (2-5) determines whether a service area covered by transit stops is selected to remain in the system. Constraint (2-6) specifies that a total of p stops are to be selected. Constraints (2-7) are integer restrictions on the decision variables.

2.4.2. Optimizing the Distribution of Bus Stop Shelters

Law and Taylor (2001) analyzed the factors affecting bus shelter placement in the Los Angeles transit system. The current shelter placement policy in Los Angeles is dictated by the potential to sell shelter advertisements and political concerns, and is only peripherally based on bus stop use. Using data on shelter and stop locations, boardings, and headways, the authors developed a methodology for measuring the cumulative use of bus stops in terms of person-minutes of wait time. Person-minutes were calculated by multiplying the number of people waiting at a stop by the average amount of time, in minutes, that they spend waiting for the bus. The final data show that bus riders were under the protection of a transit shelter only during 20 percent of the time they spent waiting for buses. After a comparison of three scenarios that optimize the goals of 1) private shelter providers, 2) locally elected officials, and 3) bus patrons, respectively, the result shows that either of the latter two scenarios would dramatically increase the time that bus patrons in Los Angeles spend sheltered while waiting for buses at stops. This analysis shows the advantage of boarding data in combination with headway data in the planning of bus stop shelter locations.

2.4.3. Uniform Density Problem in GIS Buffer Analysis

Zhao *et al.* (1998) pointed out that the results of the buffer method analysis, traditionally based on population and employment, were evenly distributed across spatial units like traffic analysis zones (TAZs), census tracts, or census block groups. Buffers around transit stops created with a given size (usually a one-quarter-mile radius) were defined as "service areas." The percentage of the population and the employed that have access to transit facilities in a zone is assumed to be the same as the ratio of the buffer area falling within the zone to the total area of the zone. However, in most cases, a zone with the same land use designation will vary somewhat in density, or it may have different land uses and significant variations in density. Zones with uniform distribution only account for a small part of most service areas. Also, the buffer method assumes that the walking distance for a transit user accessing a transit stop is the same as the Euclidian distance (straight line or air distance). The actual walking distance to a transit stop depends on the real-world street configuration, or if any streets or walking paths connect the residence to the transit stop. Furthermore, barriers and obstacles prevent people with disabilities from accessing transit facilities. The same problem occurs when measuring the effect of overlapping service areas on passenger boardings at bus stops. Instead of uniform density, street density, number of dwelling units in a parcel database, barriers to walking, and utilized network distance were introduced in transit stop accessibility analyses.

Despite these limitations, a one-quarter-mile walking distance is a well-known rule of thumb for planning public transit service and selecting bus stop locations. In most real cases, bus stops are spaced closer than a quarter mile, creating overlapping bus stop service areas on the same route. In many areas, parallel bus routes are spaced at distances less than one-half mile, creating overlapping service areas between routes that often operate at different service frequencies. To analyze and control for these overlapping service areas, a model that uses geographic information systems (GIS) analysis is used to measure the accessibility of each parcel to bus stops within walking distance as well as the integral accessibility of each bus stop to dwelling units within walking distance to the stop. The distance decay parameters in the accessibility measure is an improvement compared to the traditional methods in which ridership is related to potential transit demand by 1) intersecting census block groups with bus stop buffers using aerial interpolation to calculate population, or 2) counting the number of housing units within stop buffers. These methods, based on the questionable assumption of uniform population density and service demand, allocate population or housing units to transit service areas.

Other than using the traditional arbitrary one-quarter-mile service area buffer, in which the probability of demand falls from one to zero at exactly a one-quarter-mile distance, Zhao *et al.* (2003) fitted the following negative exponential function to survey data showing walking distance to transit stops:

$$p = e^{-6.864d_{ij}} \qquad (2\text{-}8)$$

where

p = the probability of demand, and
d = distance from facility i to the transit stop j.

Kimpel *et al.* (2007) proposed the following negative logistic function based on the Portland bus system:

$$p = \frac{e^{(a-b\cdot d_{ij})}}{1 + e^{(a-b\cdot d_{ij})}} \qquad (2\text{-}9)$$

where

p = the probability of demand,
a = intercept parameter,
b = slope parameter, and
d_{ij} = distance from facility i to the transit stop j.

This model was suited for the distance decay of transit demand to reflect a more gradual decline in transit demand at shorter distances, a steeper decline as distance approaches one-quarter mile, and a more gradual tail. The authors also tested different combinations of intercept parameter a and slope parameter b, and compared with Zhao *et al.*'s exponential function exp(-6.864d), as well as the uniform density of demand assumption (UDD), where p = 1 for d <= 0.25 miles and p = 0 for d > 0.25 miles (Table 2-7). Figure 2-2 shows this information graphically. The authors concluded that parameters a = 2 and b = 15 were the best representation of distance decay using the negative logistic function since this particular model provided the best fit to real data. This parameter set depicted steep distance decay prior to one-quarter mile. The probability of taking the bus is higher at short walking distances, and the probability is close to 0.1 at distances approaching one-quarter mile.

The above research illustrates the power of analysis using available detailed disaggregate data, boardings at the bus stop level, and parcel level counts of dwelling units. A GIS analysis was needed to relate dwelling units to the street network and to calculate distances to bus stops. A distance decay function was derived and used to compute an accessibility measure to account for overlapping bus stop service areas and improved estimation of stop-level transit demand.

Table 2-7 Estimated Probabilities for Various Distance Decay Functions (Kimpel *et al.*, 2007).

Parameters/ Distance	Negative Logistic					Negative Exponential	Uniform Density
	5-23d	4-21d	3-22d	2-22d	2-15d	-6.864d	UDD
d = 0.10 mile	0.9370	0.8699	0.6900	0.4502	0.6225	0.5034	1.0000
d = 0.20 mile	0.5987	0.4502	0.1978	0.0832	0.2689	0.2534	1.0000
d = 0.25 mile	0.3208	0.2227	0.0759	0.0293	0.1480	0.1798	1.0000
d = 0.30 mile	0.1301	0.0911	0.0266	0.0100	0.0759	0.1276	0.0000
d = 0.40 mile	0.0148	0.0121	0.0030	0.0011	0.0180	0.0642	0.0000

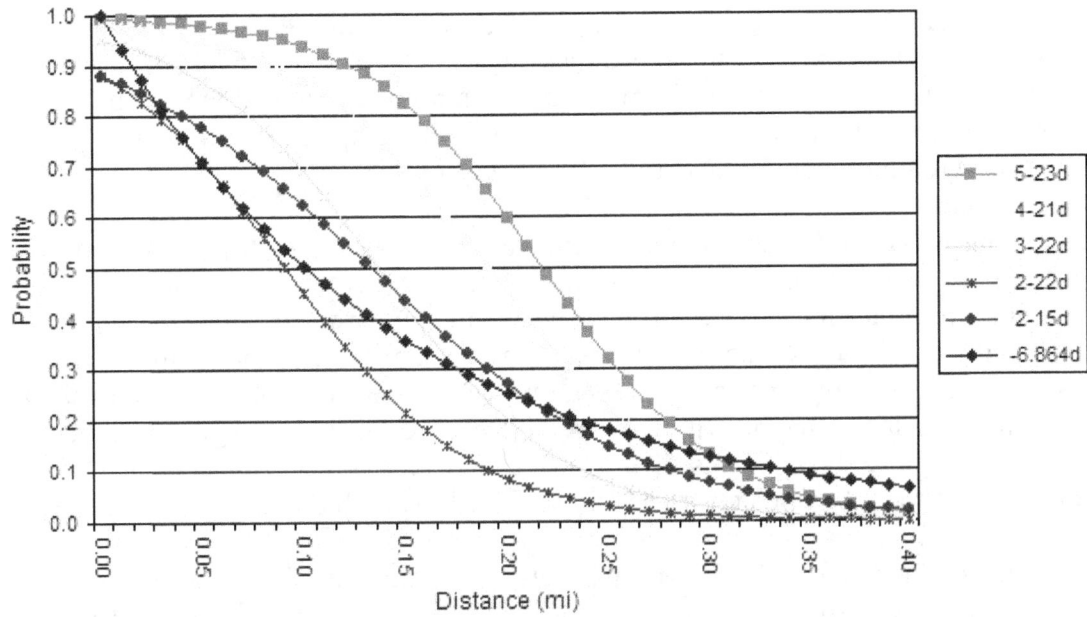

Figure 2-2 Estimated Demand Probabilities (Kimpel *et al.*, 2007).

2.5. Spatial Multicriteria Decision Making

2.5.1. Definition and Historical Background

Multicriteria analysis is a mathematical decision support tool that compares different alternatives or scenarios based on different criteria and constraints in order to help the decision makers take a more reasonable and judicious choice (Roy, 1996). Spatial multicriteria decision making (MCDM) (Thill, 1999) is an application of multicriteria analysis in a spatial context where alternatives, various criteria, and other elements of the decision problem have specific spatial dimensions. Since the late 1980s and early 1990s, spatial multicriteria analysis has been applied to real-world scenarios with the development of GIS. MCDMs have been used in a wide range of areas, such as environmental and urban planning, resource allocation and management, road planning, vehicle routing, and scheduling, as well as dealing with land suitability problems in transportation applications.

2.5.2. General Framework of Multicriteria Analysis Methods

Multicriteria methods are generally categorized as discrete and continuous. The discrete method deals with a finite, usually limited, number of pre-specified alternatives. The continuous method treats variable decision values to be determined in a continuous or integer domain of a large number (or infinite number) of choices. Figure 2-3 gives the general framework for spatial multicriteria decision analysis (Malczewski, 1999).

In the intelligence phase, the decision maker should determine the problem, which can be defined as the difference between the ideal and the existing states of the entire system. After identifying the decision problem, spatial multicriteria analysis sets evaluation criteria (objectives and attributes). This is divided into two steps. The first step is to establish a comprehensive set of objectives regarding the problem as defined. The second is to find the measures (attributes) that will measure those objectives. Using these measures, the degree to which the objectives have been achieved is used to compare alternatives. Constraints represent the natural or artificial limitations on potential alternatives. During this phase, GIS is applied to integrate all criteria and constraints for multicriteria decision analysis (Malczewski, 1999).

The second phase is called the design phase. An overall assessment method is developed for each possible alternative in this phase. Alternatives should be generated based on the set of criteria and constraints from the first phase. All the criteria are standardized with the same or a similar scale (for example, all the evaluation dimensions may be rescaled from 0 to 1), which allows comparisons for criteria among alternatives. In many multicriteria problems, the decision maker will assign weights for different criteria to reflect each criterion's relative importance to the design. During the last stage of this phase, a decision rule is used to evaluate the efficiency among alternatives to rank which alternative is preferred to another (Malczewski, 1999).

Sensitivity analysis and recommendations are included in the final phase, called the choice phase. After ranking the alternatives, sensitivity analysis is used to identify how input (geographical data and the decision maker's preference) changes affect the outputs (ranking among alternatives). If the changes do not significantly affect the outputs, the ranking is considered to be robust. On the other hand, if the result is unsatisfactory, the output must return to the evaluation criteria step and the alternatives are re-evaluated. This procedure will help decision makers learn how the various decision elements interact to determine the most preferred alternative, as well as which elements are important sources of disagreement among decision makers. After sensitivity analysis, the set of alternatives will be listed from best to worst with the same standards, and recommendations will be presented to decision makers in terms of implementing the best alternative or a set of alternatives. All of the solutions will be presented in both geographical space and criterion outcome space (Malczewski, 1999).

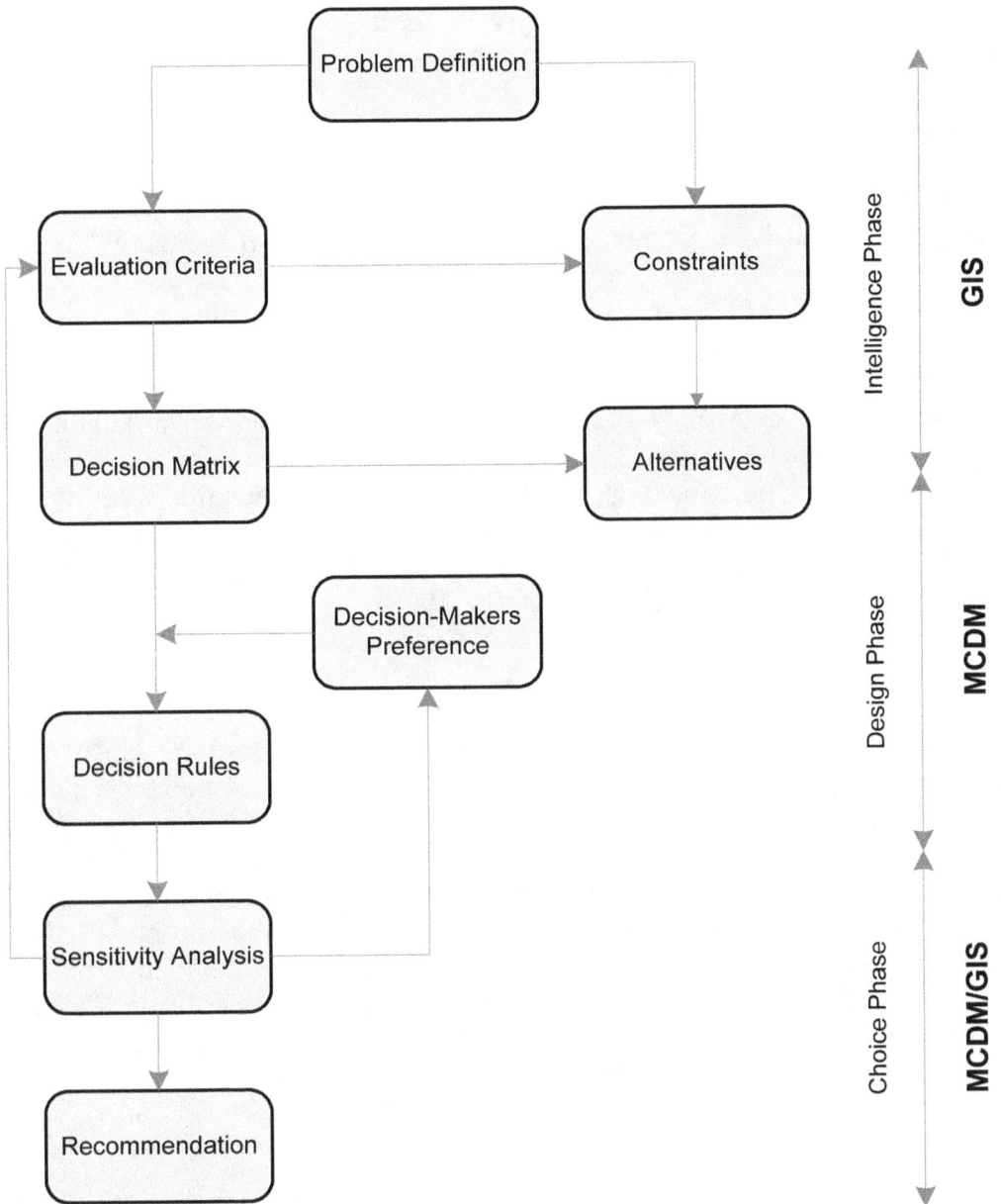

Figure 2-3 Framework for Spatial Multicriteria Decision Analysis (Malczewski, 1999).

2.5.3. Problem Definition

Any decision-making process starts with the recognition and definition of the decision problem. The decision problem is a perceived difference between the desired (or ideal) and existing states of a system. The decision maker must recognize and work to reconcile the "gap" between the desired and existing states. The intelligence phase involves searching the decision environment for data that will accurately address the problem. Raw data are obtained, processed, and examined to validate problems. The integrated GIS tools for data storage, management, manipulation, and analysis can provide major support in the problem definition stage (Malczewski, 1999).

2.5.4. Evaluation Criteria

After identifying the decision problem, the spatial multicriteria analysis sets evaluation criteria (objectives and attributes). This is divided into two steps. The first step is to establish a comprehensive set of objectives regarding the problem definition. The second is to find the measures (attributes) that will determine if the corresponding objectives have been achieved.

In a spatial context, many evaluation criteria are associated with geographical or related entities that can be represented as a map. This includes two different types of maps: the evaluation criterion map and the constraint map. The evaluation criterion map is a unique geographical attribute of alternative decisions, and is primarily used to evaluate the performance of the alternatives. The constraint map displays the limitations on the value that attributes and decision variables may assume. GIS data-handling and analysis tools are usually used to generate inputs to spatial multicriteria decision analysis (Malczewski, 1999).

2.5.5. Alternatives

Decision alternatives can be defined as alternative courses of action from which the decision maker must choose. A spatial decision alternative consists of at least two elements: action (what to do) and location (where to do it). The spatial component of a decision alternative can be deterministic, probabilistic, or linguistic. Each alternative is assigned a decision variable. The decision maker uses the variables to measure the performance of alternative decisions. Spatial decision alternatives may be discrete or continuous. A discrete method problem will involve a discrete set of pre-defined decision alternatives. Spatial alternatives are then modeled through one or a combination of the basic spatial primitives by point, line, or polygon. The continuous method problem corresponds to a high or infinite number of decision alternatives, often defined in terms of constraints (Malczewski, 1999).

2.5.6. Constraints

Constraints represent the natural or artificial restrictions on the potential alternatives. Constraints are often used in pre-analysis steps to divide alternatives into two subsets: "acceptable" or "unacceptable." An alternative will be acceptable if its performance on one criterion or several criteria can satisfy a minimum request or does not exceed a maximum limit (Chakhar, 2007).

In practice, constraints are often modeled by elementary multicriteria methods like conjunctive or disjunctive aggregation procedures. With the conjunctive method, a minimal satisfaction level $\hat{g}_j$ is associated with each criterion g_j. If the performance of an alternative with respect to different criteria is equal to or better than these minimal satisfaction levels [i.e., $g_j(a_i) > g_j$, $\forall j \in F$], the alternative is considered acceptable. Otherwise, the alternative is considered unacceptable. With the disjunctive method, the alternative is considered acceptable if it exceeds at least one satisfaction level (Chakhar, 2007).

2.5.7. Standardization

The evaluation of alternatives may face different scales (ordinal, interval, and ratio). However, multicriteria methods require that all of their criteria be expressed in the same or a similar scale. Standardizing criteria therefore rescales all of the evaluation dimensions from 0 to 1 to allow comparisons among alternatives based on the entirety of the criteria scores. In all of the vast variety of standardization procedures, standardized scores start from an initial vector $[g_j(a_1),g_j(a_2),...,g_j(a_m)]$ to obtain a standardized vector $(r_{1j},r_{2j},...,r_{mj})$ with $0< r_{ij}<1$, $\forall j \in F$, and $i = 1, ..., n$ (n being the number of alternatives). The most common standardization procedure in the multicriteria decision-making process is the linear transformation procedure. It is associated with each alternative a_i, and, for each criterion g_j, the percentage of the maximum over all alternatives (Chakhar, 2007):

$$r_{ij} = \frac{g_j(a_i)}{\max_i g_j(a_i)} \quad i = 1..., \text{n}; \ j \in F \tag{2-10}$$

where

r_{ij} = the standardized vector, and
$g_j(a_i)$ = the initial vector.

2.5.8. Criteria Weights

In many multicriteria problems, the decision maker determines that certain criteria are more important than others. This relative importance is usually expressed in terms of numbers, often called weights, which are assigned to different criteria. These weights deeply influence the final output. In extreme cases, weights will result in a non-applicable decision because the artificially determined weights are unreasonable or prejudicial. Many direct weighting techniques have been developed to help decision makers set the criteria in a specific order of preference. The cardinal "simple arrangement technique" evaluates each criterion according to a pre-established scale. Other indirect methods are also available, such as the interactive estimation method, the indifference trade-offs technique, and the analytic hierarchy process (Malczewski, 1999).

2.5.9. Decision Rules

A decision rule is the procedure by which a judgment of the efficiency among alternatives, based on the scoring order of the alternatives, determines which alternative is preferred to the others. Decision rules usually consider the context of deterministic, probabilistic, or fuzzy decisions. The main method includes the simple additive weighting method, value/utility function approaches, the analytic hierarchy process, etc. Specifically, the decision space is ordered by means of a one-to-one or one-to-many relationship of outcomes to decision alternatives. In other words, the consequences of implementing a certain alternative are given (a one-to-one relationship) or the consequences of implementing a certain alternative are uncertain (a one-to-many relationship). A "consequence" is the result of the decision—the different sets of decision consequences form the decision outcome space. Because a decision rule provides an ordering of all alternatives according to their performance and consequences related to the set of evaluation criteria, the decision problem depends on the selection of the best outcome and the identification of the decision alternative yielding this outcome or outcomes (Malczewski, 1999).

2.5.10. Sensitivity Analysis

After the ranking of alternatives, sensitivity analysis is used to identify how input changes in terms of geographical data or the decision maker's preference can affect the outputs that determine the rank of the alternatives. As mentioned previously, if the changes do not affect the outputs significantly, the ranking is treated as robust. On the other hand, if the result is unsatisfactory, the output must return to the evaluation criteria step and is re-evaluated. This procedure will help decision makers learn how the various decision elements interact to determine the most preferred alternative, as well as which elements are important sources of disagreement among decision makers (Malczewski, 1999)

2.5.11. Recommendations

Multicriteria analysis recommendations should be based on the ranking of alternatives and sensitivity analysis. Implementation of any alternative or set of alternatives should be based on these recommendations. The set of alternatives will be listed from best to worst with the same standards. All of the solutions should be presented in both geographical space and criterion outcome space (Malczewski, 1999).

2.5.12. Applications of Spatial Multicriteria Decision Making

Zhu *et al.* (2005) developed a GIS integrated multicriteria analysis model to evaluate accessibility for a housing development in Singapore. This analysis included criteria related to convenient access to public transport, community facilities, and amenities, with priorities elicited from local residents. The framework of the Zhu *et al.* analysis (see Figure 2-4) involved two major projects: a questionnaire and accessibility analysis. Through the questionnaire, Zhu *et al.* solicited opinions about the criteria for housing accessibility to given facilities (public transport, shopping centers, hospitals, or parks). After that, each facility's accessibility was assessed and ranked. The standardized accessibility assessments were put into GIS data layers, and each layer was assigned a weight derived using a multicriteria analysis technique based on questionnaire results. These data layers were then synthesized into one data layer by applying Equation (2-11) through map algebra. The output provided scores for the overall accessibility afforded by each potential location for the housing development (Malczewski, 1999):

$$score = \sum_{i=1}^{k} w_i \times s_{ij} \tag{2-11}$$

where
k = the number of criteria,
j = the alternative j under consideration,
w_j = the weight representing the relative importance of criterion i, and
s_{ij} = the score representing the relative attainment of alternative j on criterion i.

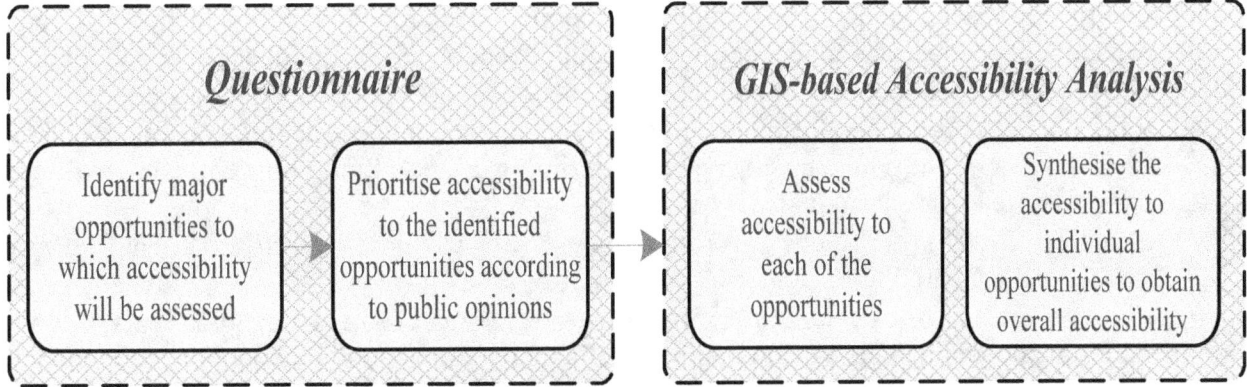

Figure 2-4 Multicriteria Framework for Accessibility Analysis.

A similar study (Moldovanyi, 2004) regarding the ranking and displaying of the marketability of pay pond businesses was implemented in West Virginia with the help of GIS and multicriteria decision making. Within this framework, the distance from a pay fishing pond to population centers, major roads, and interchangeable competition (i.e., other pay ponds and public fishing locations) are the criteria that influence marketability; these were mainly treated as evaluation criteria. For each evaluation criterion, an appropriate spatial data layer was selected for analysis. Spatial data were overlaid and queried using a buffer wizard and the straight-line distance function of the spatial analyst within GIS to obtain values for evaluation criteria. Raw data were standardized to comparable units using a field calculator and combined to create an index of marketability for each pay pond business. Each business was assigned a rank (i.e., poor, fair, moderate, good, exceptional) based on natural breaks in index scores. The results ranked a total of 32 pay ponds into five marketability levels (from highest to lowest). The results indicated that pay pond businesses should take advantage of their proximity to nearby population centers and major roads. It was also shown that shorter distances between the pay pond businesses and interchangeable competition have a negative effect on marketability.

2.6. Application Software

2.6.1. Spatial Analyst in ArcGIS

As a commonly used geographic decision support system, ArcGIS has emerged as a useful computer-based tool for spatial description and manipulation. Analysts will benefit by applying spatial operators to GIS data in order to derive new information. Among the three main types of GIS data—raster, vector, and tin—the raster data structure provides the richest modeling environment and operators for spatial analysis. The ArcGIS Spatial Analyst extension adds a comprehensive and wide range of cell-based GIS operators to ArcGIS for all spatial modeling and geoprocessing. The five major applications of the ArcGIS Spatial Analyst are (ESRI, 2007):

- *Derive new information.* Apply the Spatial Analyst tools to generate more useful information (such as watershed delineation) to classify, derive distances from roads, or calculate population density.

- *Identify spatial relationships.* Explore and compare relationships between layers through weighted overlays and combinations. Spatial Analyst also provides a rich set of map algebra tools for cell-based modeling.
- *Find suitable locations.* Find locations or areas that are most suitable for particular objectives by combining layers (such as building a new shopping center or analyzing high-risk areas for earthquakes).
- *Calculate travel cost.* According to an analysis of economic and environmental effects, travel cost is created to design optimum routes.
- *Work with all cell-based GIS data.* Regardless of the raster format, Spatial Analyst allows the user to combine cell-based GIS in specific analyses.

2.6.2. ActiveX Control in ArcGIS

The optimization model is usually developed using Visual Basic for Applications (VBA) code or another general computer language code. These codes are mainly dependent on ESRI ActiveX control (map object control) as added to a regular VBA format in an Excel macro environment (VBA editor) (ESRI, 2002).

Microsoft Visual Basic (VB) is an event-driven programming language and an associated development environment created by Microsoft. VB enables rapid application development (RAD) of graphical user interface (GUI) applications, access to databases, and creation of ActiveX controls. ESRI has adopted Visual Basic as its main programming tool. The new version of Visual Basic has been tailored to accommodate ESRI programming objects (e.g., map, polygon, point, etc.) and is known as ArcGIS Visual Basic for Application (ESRI, 2002).

An ActiveX control is a component program object that can be used by multiple programs. ActiveX controls could be considered add-ins to Microsoft Visual Basic, and they enrich the programming tools provided by Microsoft Visual Basic. ESRI has introduced different ActiveX controls that could be incorporated with Microsoft Visual Basic and Microsoft Office Visual Basic for Application (Microsoft VBA) (ESRI, 2002).

2.6.3. Transit Stop Inventory Collecting Tool

The Automated Transit Stop Inventory Model (ATSIM) is a user-friendly mobile-desktop system designed to collect, update, and analyze standard transit stop inventories for transit agencies in Florida (LCTR 2007). The mobile component of ATSIM consists of a PDA application designed for the easy data entry of transit stop information in the field, which include Global Positioning System (GPS) and a built-in digital camera (see Figures 2-5 and 2-6). The system allows for the collection of 56 standard attributes, in addition to one general comment field, six user-defined fields, two GPS location fields (latitude and longitude), and multiple digital photos at each stop.

Another advantage, ATSIM is fully combined within the GIS function. ATSIM makes use of the following two types of files: an Extensible Markup Language (XML) file used by the PDA field collection system and shape files used by its GIS component. ATSIM provides a conversion function that can convert the bus stop inventory in the PDA to standard GIS shape files. According to the integrated GIS interface, users can easily retrieve bus stop attributes and pictures, quickly query the bus stop inventory with reference to a specific set of features, and generate a summary table and chart as well (for example, to calculate the percentage of bus stops not accessible to riders with disabilities).

With ATSIM, the following ADA-related attributes will be easy to inventory:

1. Loading Pads: Whether there is a loading pad to load people in wheelchairs.
2. Obstructions: Whether there are obstructions that will prevent people in wheelchairs from accessing the stop, including obstructions in any access direction.
3. Curb Cuts: Whether the stop includes ramps to allow people in wheelchairs to get to the transit stop.
4. Nearby Pedestrian Crossing: Whether there is a nearby pedestrian crossing that may be used by people in wheelchairs.
5. Terrain: Whether the general terrain is Flat, Minor Slope, and Major Slope (standard selections).
6. Surface: Whether the immediate floor surface of the stop is Mostly Concrete, Mostly Brick, Mostly Wood, Mostly Gravel, Mostly Grass, Mostly Soil/Sand, or Other (standard selections).
7. ADA: Whether the stop meets one of three levels of ADA accessibility: Accessible, Functional, and Not Accessible. A transit stop is considered accessible when persons in wheelchairs can access it. Persons in wheelchairs can access functional stops, but the stop may not be in full compliance with ADA regulations. A stop is considered inaccessible if persons in wheelchairs cannot reach it.

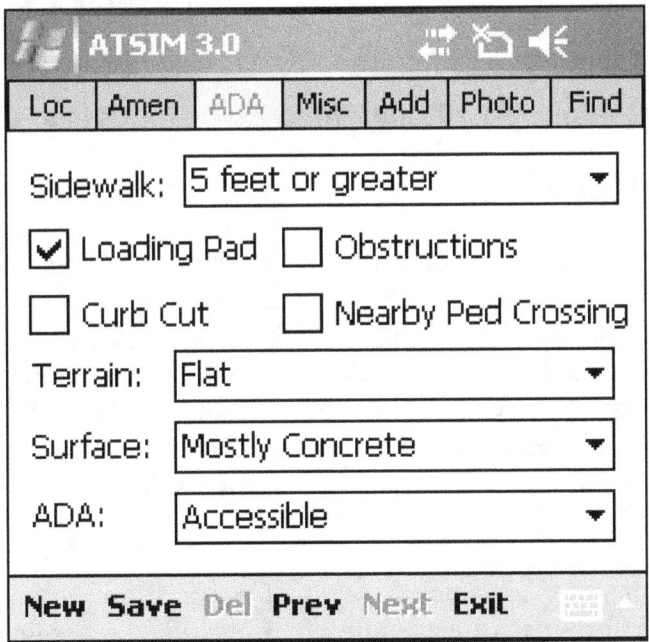

Figure 2-5 Data Entry Screen for ADA-Related Amenities.

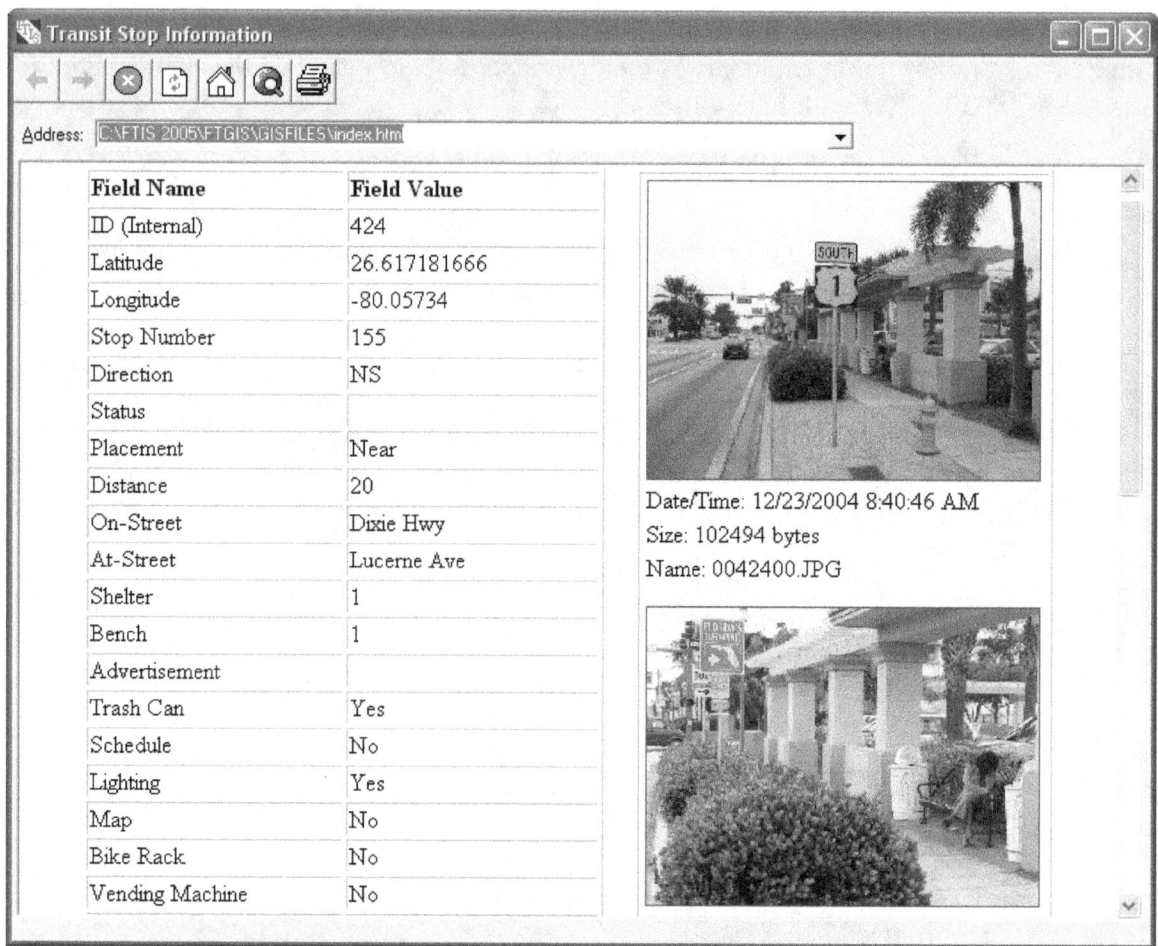

Figure 2-6 Retrieved Transit Stop Attribute Data and Pictures.

2.6.4 LINGO/LINDO API

The LINGO/LINDO Application Programming Interface (API) is among the most famous optimization software for use in operational research. It was developed by LINDO Systems, Inc. As the first nonlinear programming software for personal computers, LINGO provides a comprehensive tool designed to make building and solving linear, nonlinear, and integer optimization models faster, easier, and more efficient. LINGO also provides a completely integrated package that includes a powerful language for expressing optimization models, a full-featured environment for building and editing problems, and a set of fast built-in problem solvers.

LINDO API enables the user to develop personal optimization applications. It integrates the LINDO problem solver formulas directly into other customized applications. At the same time, LINDO API runs as a MATLAB external function, and uses MATLAB's modeling and programming environment to build and solve models and create custom algorithms based on the LINDO API's routines and solvers.

2.7. Summary

In this chapter, a comprehensive literature search and review has been performed to investigate the accessibility standards from ADA and university design for bus stops, public transit pattern study for people with disabilities, current research on spatial multicriteria decision making and the application software.

The Americans with Disabilities Act (ADA) of 1990 provided guidelines and minimum requirements regarding bus stop accessibility for persons with disabilities. Transit agencies must adhere to these requirements during new construction and improvements to existing facilities. The major concern of the ADA minimum requirements is to ensure that a given bus stop can provide adequate connections to the bus stop, as well as to enable boarding and disembarking for riders with disabilities. It focused on satisfying specific minimum technical criteria to allow most people with disabilities to use the built environment. By contrast, universal design concepts intend to provide a more comfortable environment than strict ADA adherence, including features like benches, shelters, lighting, etc., that additionally make the experience better for all transit users.

Most bus stop accessibility research has focused on bus stop location optimization, which is different from the focus on fixed-route bus stops in this research. However, some ideas presented in previous research are useful for the purposes of this study. One example is the location set covering problem (LSCP) model, which seeks to minimize the number of stops in one analysis region within which there will be at least one transit stop. Another example is the maximal covering location problem (MCLP) model that is used to maximize bus stop coverage from the standpoint of location. Also valuable to this research is the Los Angeles study which investigated and summarized the relationship between ridership, wait time, and the distribution of bus stop shelters. Likewise, the research on bus transit accessibility for people with reduced mobility provides a detailed list of measurable variables that can be treated as a reliable reference.

As a major potential approach for this study, spatial multicriteria decision making and its applications in transportation problems were fully reviewed. The entire framework and methodology, its objectives, and evaluation systems were found to be suitable for this research. Spatial analysis and the ActiveX interface of ArcGIS were introduced as they relate to the programming of optimization models.

CHAPTER 3

METHODOLOGY

This chapter first provides an overview of the general methodology for developing optimization models that aim to identify a list of bus stops for accessibility improvements. The models will attempt to maximize the benefits to riders with disabilities given an available annual budget for such improvements. In support of the methodology, this chapter also describes the main data resources to be used, an analytical hierarchy process (AHP) for combining qualitative and quantitative factors, and the method to be used for optimization model development.

3.1. Methodology Overview

To develop a feasible bus stop multicriteria optimization model that can be used to study accessibility for riders with disabilities, the following major steps are necessary, as depicted in Figure 3-1:

1) Develop a full requirement checklist to evaluate current bus stop conditions for riders with disabilities based on the ADA minimum requirements and universal design elements. This bus stop checklist will be used for a bus stop field survey that will provide the major constraints for use in the optimization models.

2) Acquire and clean various transit and socioeconomic data to construct evaluation criteria for multicriteria optimization models. The types of data will include:

   - Data that describe the distribution and various classifications of the subpopulations with disabilities throughout the community.
   - The "worker flow" tables that provide information about disability status, age, and means of transportation to work.
   - Basic bus service information including stop location, stop interval, bus schedule, and headway.
   - Ridership or Automatic Passenger Counter (APC) results based on routes or stops if they are available.
   - Bus stop connectivity information (e.g., sidewalks).
   - Land use information (i.e., industry, hospital, recreational facility, etc.).
   - An existing bus stop inventory.
   - Data that describe bus service system operation, maintenance, and budget information.

3) Create a suitable service buffer radius for riders with disabilities. The bus stop service radius is generally considered to be approximately one-quarter mile (400 meters), although less urbanized areas and areas that have low population density generally have a larger bus stop service radius. Given that the mobility of riders with disabilities is lower than that of average riders, the actual service buffer radius for the riders with disabilities should be lower than one-quarter mile. Likewise, coherent connectivity to the bus stop is more important to riders with disabilities.

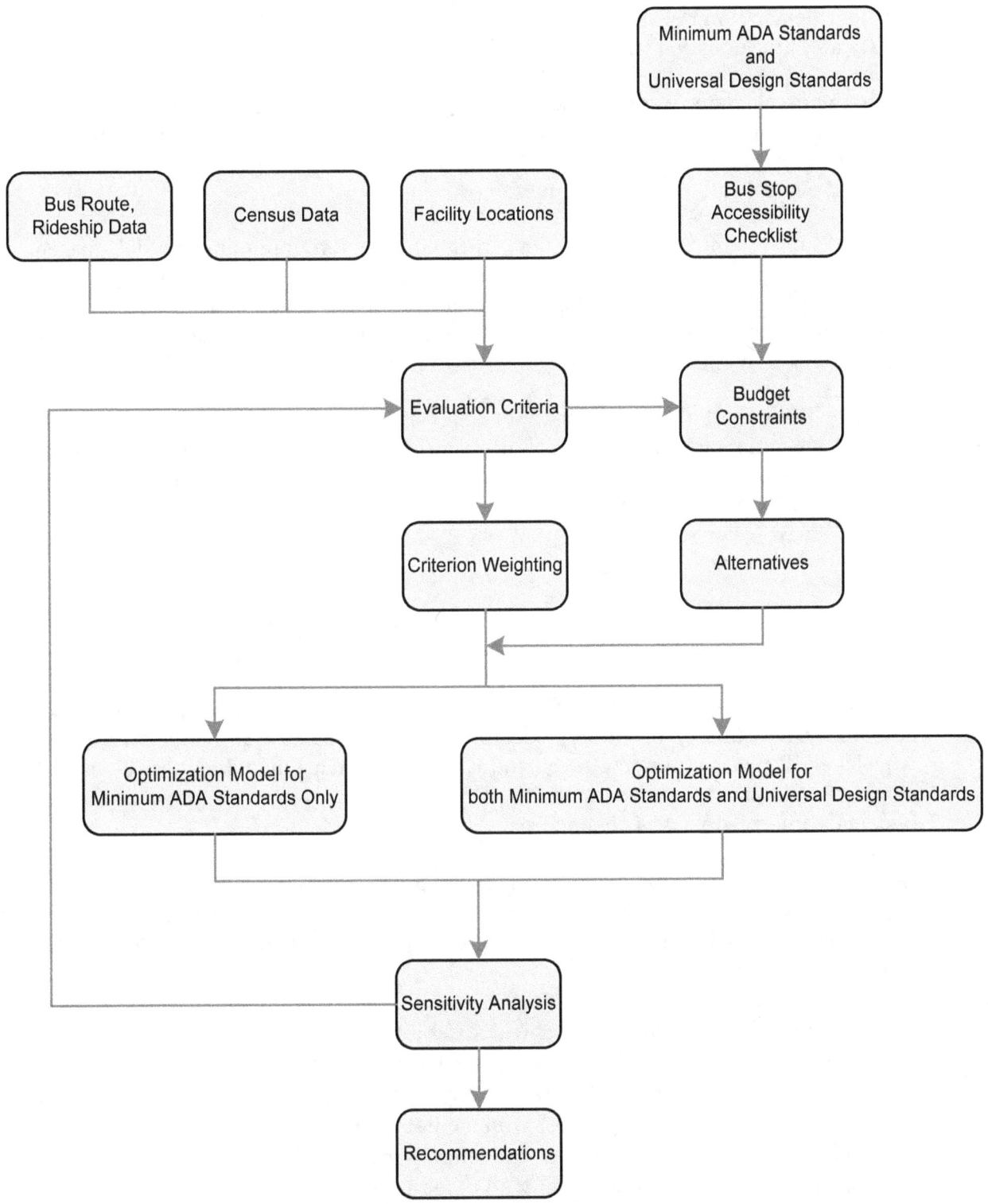

Figure 3-1 Framework for Model Development.

4) Determine constraints and feasible alternatives. Transit agency operational and maintenance budgets will be treated as the main constraints. Other formulations might

consider demand and cost elasticities. A feasible alternatives list must be developed to satisfy all of the constraints.

5) Assign and calculate weights based on evaluation criteria. Every criterion has its own evaluation unit(s) and standard evaluation(s), such as economic and environmental or qualitative and quantitative. An analytical hierarchy process (AHP) will be introduced to rank and evaluate all of the alternatives.

6) Develop an optimization model. As a goal, the programming model, based on multicriteria spatial analysis, is developed to maximize the overall benefits to patrons with disabilities from transit stop improvements. The mathematical formulation will capture the best solution among different types of improvements and among different locations based on budgetary, equity, and feasibility constraints.

7) Evaluate the output through sensitivity analysis. Sensitivity analysis is conducted to validate the rationality and influence of criteria on the criterion weights and criterion (attribute) values. Based on the results, conclusions and recommendations can be made regarding the optimization models.

3.2. Available Data Sources

The data sources available for this research include those from the Broward County Mass Transit (BCT) and the U.S. Census Bureau. They are detailed below.

1. *Broward County Mass Transit (BCT)*: Available databases from BCT currently include a comprehensive bus stop inventory, a detailed ridership database at the transit stop level, a wheelchair database at the stop level, and various GIS maps including bus routes and bus stops. In addition, documentation of all of the improvement contracts, as well as budgetary information, was obtained.

2. *Census Blockgroup 2000*: The data describing the distribution of Broward County's population with disabilities will be extracted or calculated from 2000 Census Summary Tape File #3, which makes the following data available at the census blockgroup and census tract levels:

   - Total population 5 years and over with disabilities
   - Total population 5 years and over with sensory disabilities
   - Total population 5 years and over with physical disabilities
   - Total population 5 years and over with mental disabilities
   - Total population 5 years and over with employment disabilities
   - Total population 5 years and over with other disabilities

3. *Census Transportation Planning Package (CTPP) 2000*: CTPP 2000 is a special tabulation of responses from households completing the Census long form. The special tabulation is used to provide data to support a wide range of transportation planning activities. It is the only Census product that summarizes data by place of work and tabulates the flow of workers from home to workplace. It is also the only source of

information with summary tabulations available for traffic analysis zones (TAZs) that have been defined by state and regional transportation agencies. This dataset includes disability status, age, and means of transportation to work. This information can be mapped according to place of residence. It is the result of a cooperative effort between various groups, including the state Department of Transportation, the U.S. Census Bureau and the Federal Highway Administration. The data were collected in 2000 and are shown at the tract level.

4. *Florida Geographic Data Library* (FGDL): FGDL is a mechanism for distributing spatial (GIS) data throughout the state of Florida. FGDL is warehoused and maintained at the University of Florida's GeoPlan Center, a GIS research and teaching facility. Currently, over 350 current and historic GIS layers from over 35 local, state, federal, and private agencies are included in the FGDL. Specifically, FGDL includes data on land use/land cover, hydrography, soils, transportation, boundaries, environmental quality, conservation, census, as well as several related attributes. FGDL also provided information on the non-household trip end, which includes workplace, hospital, shopping mall, recreational facility, and other location information.

3.3. Analytic Hierarchy Process

The analytical hierarchy process (AHP) is a multicriteria decision technique that can combine qualitative and quantitative factors for prioritizing, ranking, and evaluating alternatives. This research uses AHP to compare and evaluate the different criteria, such as the distribution of persons with disabilities, ridership, and land use, and then assign weights to them. The first step in AHP is to develop a hierarchical representation of a problem. At the top of the hierarchy is the overall objective. The decision alternatives are at the bottom. Between the top and bottom levels are the relevant attributes of the decision problem for comparing alternatives. In the GIS application, the alternatives are represented in GIS databases, and each layer contains the attribute values assigned to the alternatives. Each alternative (e.g., cell or polygon) is related to the higher-level elements (i.e., attributes). The attribute concept links the AHP method to GIS-based procedures. The number of levels in the hierarchy depends on the complexity of the problem and the decision maker's model of the problem hierarchy. Once the hierarchical representation is identified, the program generates relational data for comparing alternatives. After determining the relative priority of each attribute using the comparisons, the program calculates the priorities or weights of the lowest-level alternatives relative to the top-most objective.

The AHP uses composite weights to represent ratings of alternatives with respect to the overall goal. The weights, also referred to as decision alternatives scores, are the basis from which decisions can be made. They serve as ratings of the effectiveness of each alternative in achieving the goal. The overall score, *R*, is defined as follows:

$$R_i = \sum_k w_k r_{ik} \qquad (3\text{-}1)$$

where
R_i = the overall score of the *i*th alternative;

w_k = the vector of priorities associated with the kth element of the criterion hierarchical structure, $\sum w_k = 1$; and

r_{ik} = the vector of priorities derived from comparing alternatives on each criterion.

The most preferred alternative is selected by identifying the maximum value of R_i. The AHP method will be illustrated using a site-suitability problem (see Figure 3-2). This problem involves evaluating three potential sites for bus stop development based on economic and environmental objectives (Malczewski, 1999). The objectives are measured in terms of three criteria: price (p), slope (s), and view (v). The overall goal is to identify the best parcel. This requires assessing the relative importance of the elements at each level of the decision hierarchy (i.e., objectives, attributes, and alternatives). The detailed GIS-based rating procedure is described in the subsections below.

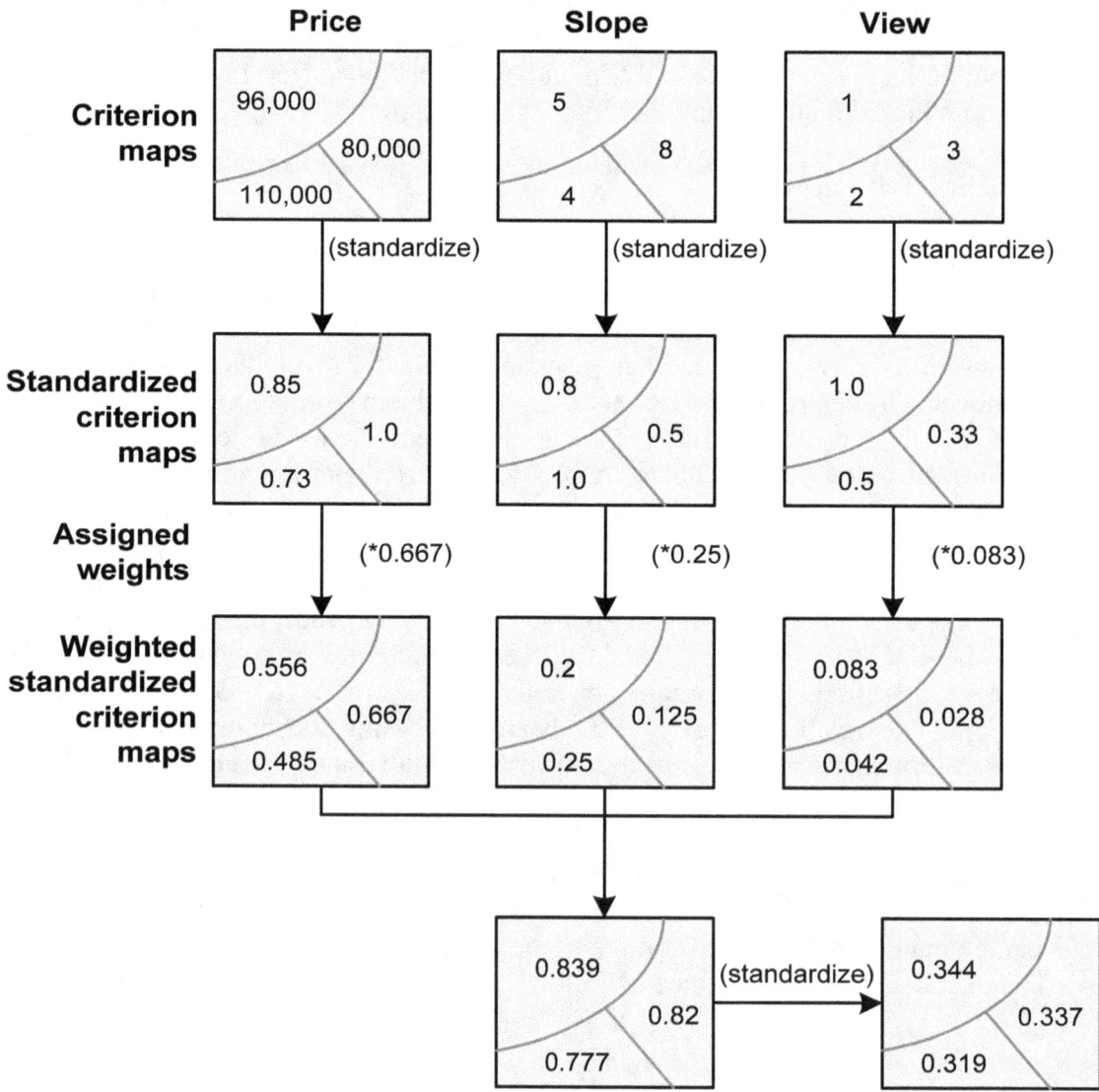

Figure 3-2 Analytic Hierarchy Process Method Procedures.

3.3.1. Standardization of Criterion Maps

In the first stage, the data layers are standardized using the equation below:

$$x'_j = \frac{x_j^{min}}{x_{ij}}$$ (3-2)

where

x'_j = the standardized value for the jth attribute,

x_j^{min} = the minimum score for the jth attribute, and

x_{ij} = the raw score.

For example, in Figure 3-2, the standardized value of 0.83 for criterion price (p) is calculated by dividing 80,000 by 96,000, and the standardized value of 0.73 is calculated by dividing 80,000 by 110,000.

3.3.2. Weighting of Standardized Criterion Maps

In the second stage, each standardized criterion map is multiplied by the corresponding weight. The weight reflects the importance among the three factors, which add to a total of 1.0. For example, if the economic factor price (p) is 0.667, and the environmental factor is 0.333, where the environmental factor includes slope and view: slope (s) is estimated to be three times more important than view (v), then slope (s) is 0.25 and view (v) is 0.083.

3.3.3. Rating of Criterion Maps

In the third and last stage, the weighted standardized criterion maps are added together by overlaying the operation to obtain a rating for all alternatives. The final rating could be standardized by dividing each value on the rating map by the sum of the total. Finally, the results show that the area ranking 0.344 is the most suitable, followed by the area ranking 0.337. The area ranking 0.319 is the least suitable for development.

3.4. Goal Programming

Among bus stop improvements for riders with disabilities, the ADA minimum requirements are the only compulsory standards. Other improvements are introduced given suitable conditions based on the universal design concepts as mentioned in Subsection 2.1.2, such as setting up shelters where a high level of bus ridership merits them. The optimization models seek to achieve these two improvements standards. Because the requirements for the two objectives are different, goal programming is introduced to satisfy them both at the same time.

Goal programming alternatives attempt to achieve goals in terms of target levels rather than quantities to be maximized or minimized. An optimal compromise among the different objectives will then be derived to minimize deviations from the goals. Whereas linear programming identifies the point that optimizes a single objective from the series of feasible solutions, goal programming determines the point that will best satisfy the series of goals in the decision problem. The goal programming approach requires the decision maker to specify the most desirable goal for each objective at the principal level.

In weighted goal programming, the objective is to find a solution that minimizes the weighted sum of the goal deviations. The objective function for this type of goal programming is expressed as:

$$\min \sum_{k} (w_k^- d_k^- + w_k^+ d_k^+) \tag{3-3}$$

where

w_k^-, w_k^+ = negative and positive weights corresponding to several goal deviations, and

d_k^-, d_k^+ = negative and positive goal deviations.

The weights represent additional information reflecting the decision maker's preferences with respect to the deviation variables. The method assumes that the positive deviations and negative deviations of the criterion outcomes from the goals are equally undesirable. That is, the decision maker perceives both overachievement and underachievement of specified goals as equally undesirable outcomes. In this case, the decision maker will act according to a strictly satisfying principle.

3.5. Summary

The methodology described in this chapter consists of three main stages. During the first stage of development, a bus stop accessibility checklist based on ADA minimum requirements is used to evaluate existing bus stops. Bus stops, transit ridership, and socioeconomic data from three main sources were collected and processed to generate evaluation criteria and alternatives. Census and Broward County Transit (BCT) data were used. BCT possesses a comprehensive bus stop inventory, a detailed ridership database at the route level, a wheelchair database at the bus stop level, various GIS maps that include bus routes and bus stops improvement contracts, and budgetary information. In addition, the 2000 Census offers information on the spatial distribution and types of populations with disabilities at the census tract and block group levels.

During the second stage, the analytical hierarchy process (AHP) is used to 1) combine qualitative and quantitative factors for prioritizing, ranking, and evaluating alternatives; 2) compare and evaluate different criteria such as the distribution of persons with disabilities, ridership, and land use; and 3) assign weights to bus stops.

In the final stage, two optimization models using the mathematical programming techniques are formulated to meet two objectives: 1) satisfying the minimum ADA standards, and 2) satisfying ADA minimum standards in combination with universal design standards. These two models seek to find the optimal total bus stop weights (combined those from all criteria considered) that maximize the overall system benefit within a limited budget. The models are formulated such that all selected bus stops can be brought into compliance with minimum ADA accessibility standards as well. Major constraints are determined based on the budget allocations for bus stop accessibility improvement and construction costs for bus stop facilities.

CHAPTER 4

DATA PREPARATION

This chapter describes the data collection and integration process. The data from all the different sources, including Broward County Transit (BCT), Florida Geographic Data Library (FGDL), and Census Transportation Planning Package (CTPP), were acquired and organized to generate evaluation criteria. A unified database integrated bus stop status and other criteria were developed in the analytical hierarchy process (AHP). The basic unit of analysis was the bus stop service area based on the street network. Furthermore, this chapter presents the ADA improvement budget of Broward County and the construction cost estimate checklist for candidate bus stops based on estimates from current contractors.

4.1. Bus Stop and Ridership Data

Broward County Transit (BCT) possesses a bus stop status inventory that includes data on 5,034 bus stops serving 43 different bus routes. This inventory includes information about all of the bus stop facilities including ADA accessibility status. In Broward County, 1,616 bus stops are only "functional" and another 849 bus stops are not accessible for physically challenged riders, for a total of 2,465 bus stops (49 percent) that do not meet minimum ADA requirements (Figure 4-1). Figure 4-2 shows the current bus stop distribution in Broward County, where dark nodes represent inaccessible bus stops and white nodes represent accessible bus stops. Because some bus routes cross the county boundary into Miami-Dade and Palm Beach Counties, a quarter-mile radius buffer along those routes was developed to maintain the integrity of the entire bus stop system. Inaccessible bus stops clearly pervade the whole bus stop system. Since 1996, BCT has been in the process of improving the accessibility of bus stops with a target of making 300-500 additional bus stops accessible each year. At this rate, BCT plans to make all prioritized bus stops accessible within the next five years.

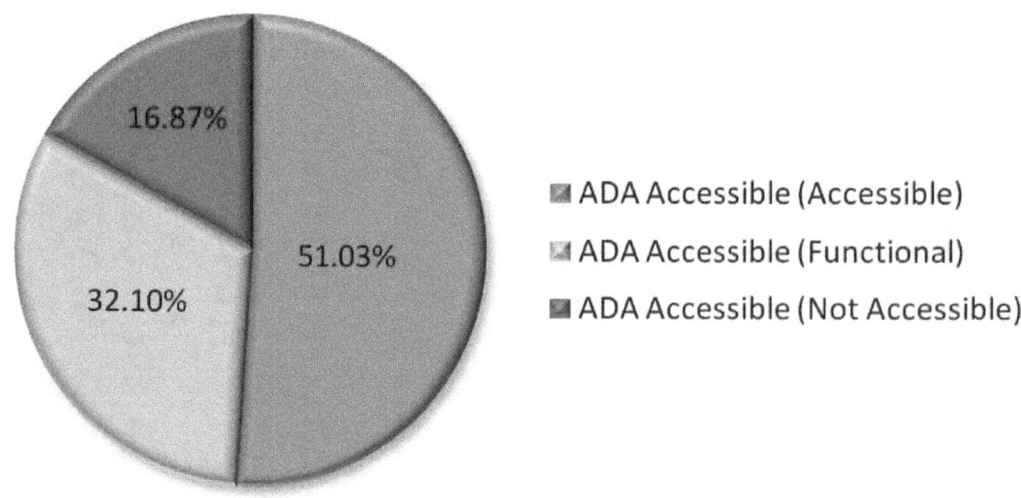

Figure 4-1 Bus Stop Accessibility in Broward County.

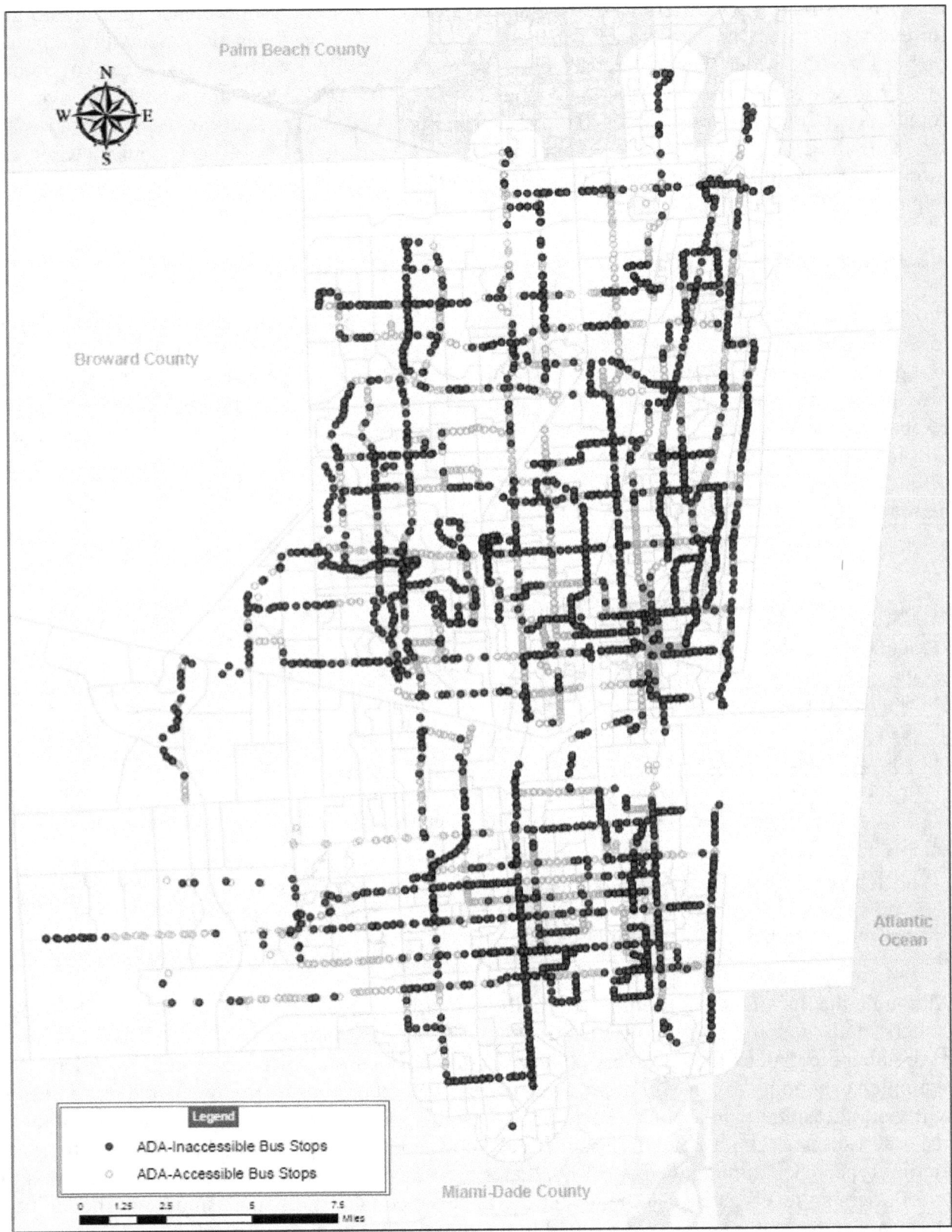

Figure 4-2 Broward County Transit Bus Stop Locations.

BCT also provides two different bus ridership datasets to weigh the importance of accessibility for every bus stop. One dataset includes the number of times wheelchair passengers board based on bus stop IDs, which were collected from March 2006 through October 2007. A total of 55 out of 289 buses used automatic passenger counters (APCs); APC buses are rotated to cover all routes. After 2008, Broward County Transit updated the APC data collection system. As a result, over one-third of the buses were equipped with APC, which ran on all bus routes. After six months' testing, ridership data for individual bus stops for the period between May 2008 and September 2008 became available.

4.2. Demographic Characteristics and Other Factors

It is important to understand the travel patterns of the population with disabilities. Origin locations and common destinations (including health care facilities like hospitals, parks, private and public schools, religious centers, and shopping centers and supermarkets) help inform transit providers as they attempt to improve services to this community (Collia *et al.*, 2003; Scottish Executive Social Research, 2006). The Florida Geographic Data Library (FGDL) provides the GIS layers explained in Table 4-1 to weight bus stops.

Table 4-1 GIS Layer Descriptions of Different Factors.

Content Title	Publisher	Feature Type	Extent	Year
Population w/ Disabilities	US Census Bureau	polygon	Broward County	2000
Health Care Facilities 2005	University of Florida GeoPlan Center	point	STATE	2005
Shopping Centers	University of Florida GeoPlan Center	point	STATE	2003
Parks	University of Florida GeoPlan Center	point	STATE	2005
Private and Public School	University of Florida GeoPlan Center	point	STATE	2008
Religious Center Facility	University of Florida GeoPlan Center	point	STATE	2005
People w/ Disabilities Work-End Flow	Census Transportation Planning Package	polygon	Broward County	2000
Wheelchair Boarding	Broward County Transit	dBASE	Broward County	03/2006-10/2007
Ridership per Stop	Broward County Transit	dBASE	Broward County	05/2008-09/2008

Although the locations of health care facilities, parks, private and public schools, religious centers, and shopping centers are not directly related to the boardings at every bus stop, they have the potential to attract riders. Every facility will attract different kinds of riders; for example, a shopping center will attract more riders than common supermarkets, and more people will visit a hospital than a clinic. Each type of facility must be evaluated separately for a more accurate estimate. Unfortunately, it is difficult to establish a realistic number of riders for each facility type. The "importance factor" evaluates the transit ridership for each facility in terms of gross ridership levels, such that the higher the importance factor, the more important the facility. Descriptions for every factor are provided in the sections below.

4.2.1. Populations with Disabilities

The residential and destination locations of populations with disabilities are the most important factors in determining which bus stops should implement ADA improvements, and when. Obviously, those areas that have a greater percentage of persons with disabilities deserve to have higher quality transit services. Hence, distribution data were extracted or calculated from the 2000 Census Summary Tape File #3, which provides data at the census blockgroup and census tract levels and includes the total population with disabilities five years of age and over within Broward County. Figure 4-3 shows the distribution of the County's population with disabilities.

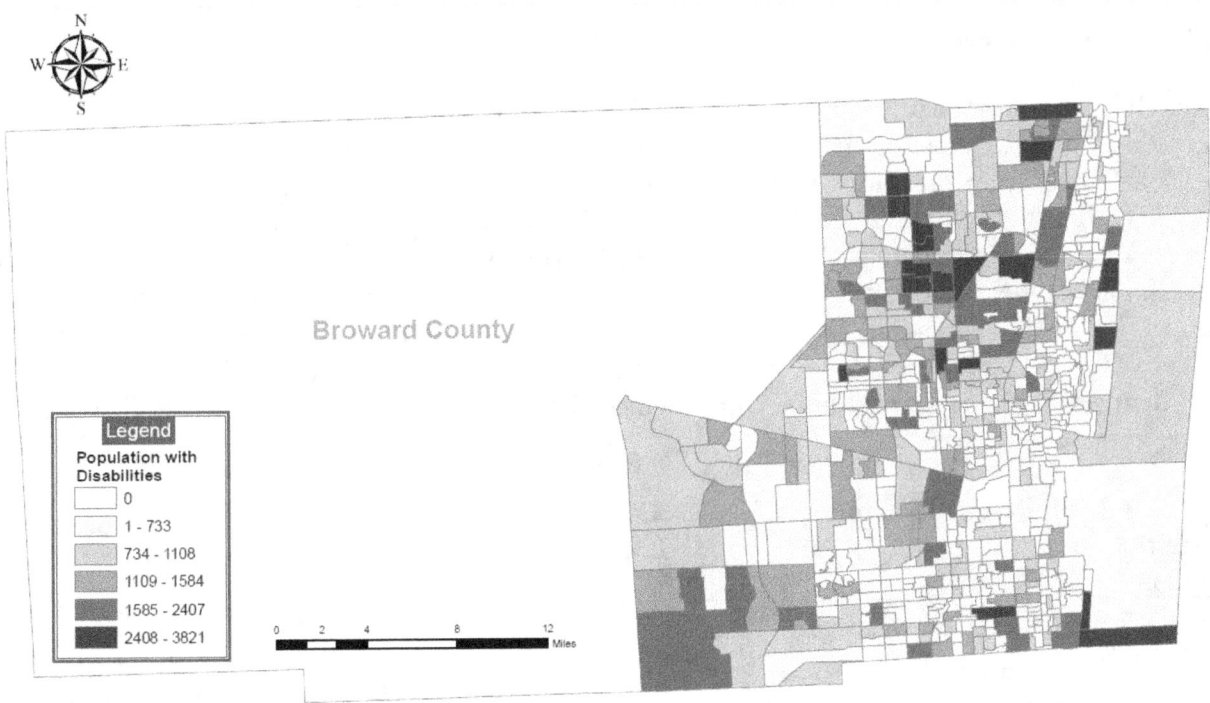

Figure 4-3 Distribution of the Population with Disabilities in Broward County.

4.2.2. Parks

The GIS layer for parks contains park type information such as campgrounds, recreational vehicle (RV) parks, playgrounds, sports and recreational facilities, and so on. The data contains fields denoting the physical address and facility type information for parks located in Florida. Table 4-2 shows a list of park types in the dataset and their importance factors. Because most people reach RV parks and campgrounds via automobile rather than transit, a lower importance factor was assigned to these parks.

Table 4-2 Importance Factors for Parks.

Parks	Importance Factor
Activity based - baseball	3
Activity based - skate park	3
Activity based - soccer	3
Activity based - tennis court	3
Golf - driving range	3
Golf course	3
Natural resource based	3
Parks and playgrounds	3
RV parks and camp grounds	1

4.2.3. Health Centers

The GIS layer for health centers contains information on health care facility types such as hospitals, clinics, Red Cross centers, and ophthalmology facilities. Health care facility addresses were gathered from the Florida Department of Health Care, Super Pages Online, and Yellow Pages Online. This dataset contains fields denoting the physical address, type, and contact information for health care facilities located in Florida. One field that describes different health care facility types was used to determine the importance factor for each type. As Table 4-3 shows, hospitals and medical centers scored the highest importance factor ratings due to their larger scale and larger area of coverage, while specialized health service facilities such as clinics and dentists have the second higher importance factor, and community health service facilities came in the third place.

Table 4-3 Importance Factors for Health Centers.

Health Centers	Importance Factor
Hospital	3
Medical center	3
Red Cross	3
Clinic	2
Residential treatment facility	2
Skilled nursing facility	2
Adult family care home	2
Dentists	2
Ophthalmology	2
Family / general practices	2
Home health agency	2
Internal medicine	2
Ambulatory surgical center	2
Assisted living facility	1
Crisis stabilization unit	1
Health care services pool	1
Homemaker & companion services	1
Hospice	1
Intermediate care facility	1
Nurse registry	1
Transitional living facility	1

4.2.4. Religious Centers

The GIS layer for religious centers contains information on the type of religious centers such as Cathedral, Temple, Synagogue, Church, and so on, which serve individuals of Christian, Islamic, Judaic, Buddhist, and other faiths. The physical addresses and contact information for religious facilities were based on data taken from the Yellow Pages Online and the Super Pages Online. The layer contains a field that describes the type of facility and was used to determine the importance factor. As an example for description purpose, Table 4-4 gives the assigned importance factors for different religious facilities.

Table 4-4 Importance Factors for Religious Centers.

Religious Centers	Importance Factor
Cathedral	3
Temple	3
Church	2
Synagogues	2
Chapel	1

4.2.5. Public and Private Schools

The GIS layer for public and private schools contains school type information including elementary school, high school, college, and university. It contains a combination of school and educational facility addresses from 68 different sources. The data contains selected fields denoting the physical address, school number, district, and contact information for schools located in Florida. The field for school enrollment provides the total number of students in attendance, which was used to determine the importance factor. Although school enrollment is a quantitative factor, it is very difficult to use this field to determine how many people with disabilities use public transit to reach specific destinations. Using standard deviations, all schools were divided into five groups based on enrollment to minimize the deviation in every group. For description purposes, Table 4-5 gives example importance factors for five levels of school enrollment for both private and public schools.

Table 4-5 Importance Factor for Public and Private Schools.

School Enrollment	Importance Factor
2258-5060	5
1567-2257	4
876-1566	3
186-875	2
0-185	1

4.2.6. Shopping Centers

The GIS layer for shopping centers contains information on all shopping center facilities from the Yellow Pages Online. This dataset contains fields denoting the physical address and contact information for shopping center facilities located in Florida. Only two groups of shopping centers are included: shopping centers and supermarkets. Because shopping centers are expected to attract a larger number of customers (including customers with disabilities) than supermarkets, Table 4-6 shows that shopping centers were assigned a higher importance factor than supermarkets.

Table 4-6 Importance Factors for Shopping Centers.

Shopping Centers	Importance Factor
Shopping centers	3
Supermarket	1

4.2.7. Work Trips by Persons with Disabilities via Bus

The CTPP 2000 provided the data regarding ridership to work by bus for the population with disabilities. In this research, transportation to work refers to the principal mode of travel that workers generally used to get from home to work during the referenced week. Data were tabulated for workers with disabilities who are 16 years old and over for members of the Armed Forces and civilians who were at work during the referenced week. People who used different means of transportation on different days of the week were asked to specify the one they used most often—that is, the greatest number of days. People who used more than one means of transportation to get to work each day were asked to report the one used for the longest distance during the work trip. The means of transportation in this study only focuses on bus trips. The data collected in Broward County and West Palm Beach County are based on Traffic Analysis Zones (TAZ); the data collected in Miami-Dade County are based on Census Block Groups. Figure 4-4 shows ridership to work by bus for people with disabilities in Broward County.

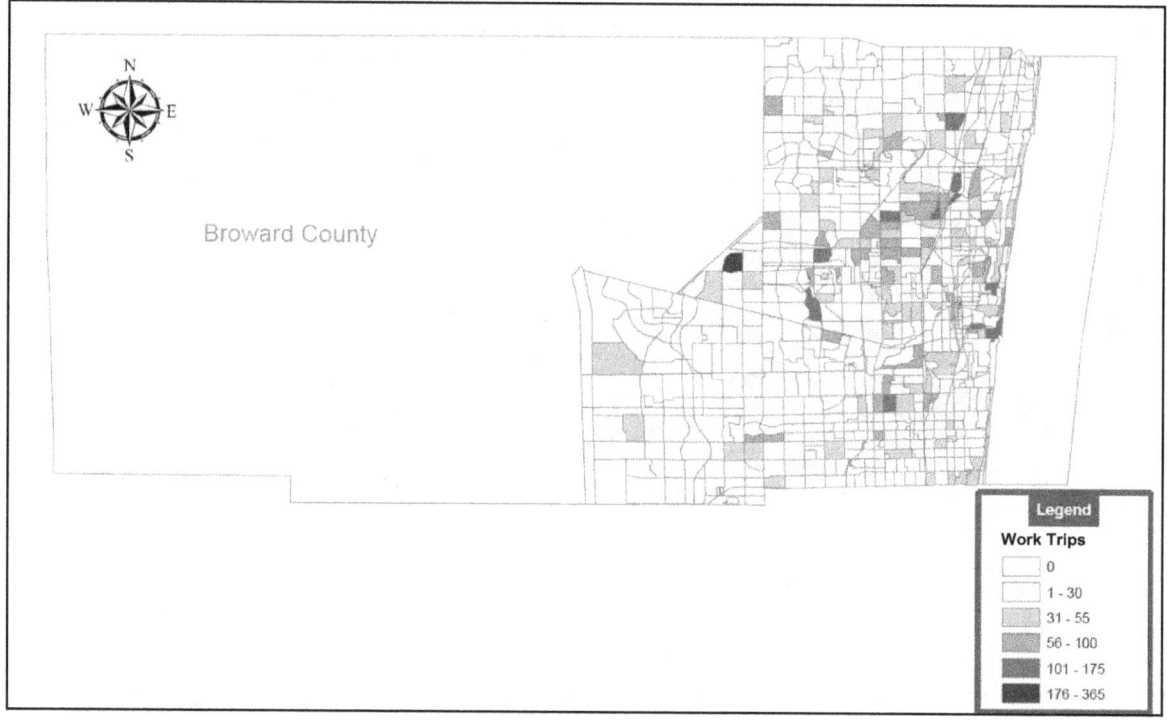

Figure 4-4 Work Trips by Persons with Disabilities in Broward County.

4.3. Service Area

To study the service scale of bus stops, the most common and easiest way is to create a "straight-line buffer"—usually with the radius of a quarter mile—around the bus stop (see the green circle in Figure 4-5). This method assumes that the walking distance to the bus stop is the Euclidian distance (a straight line). The actual walking distance depends on the real-world street configuration. Figure 4-5 shows an example involving a church located within the straight-line buffer. The Euclidian distance from this church to the bus stop is 0.23 miles, compared to the actual walking distance of 0.72 miles based on the actual street configuration. In the latter case, the distance is far beyond the standard quarter-mile service distance. It can thus be seen that service buffer area based on the actual street network (i.e., the dark irregular area in Figure 4-5) is most desirable for this analysis.

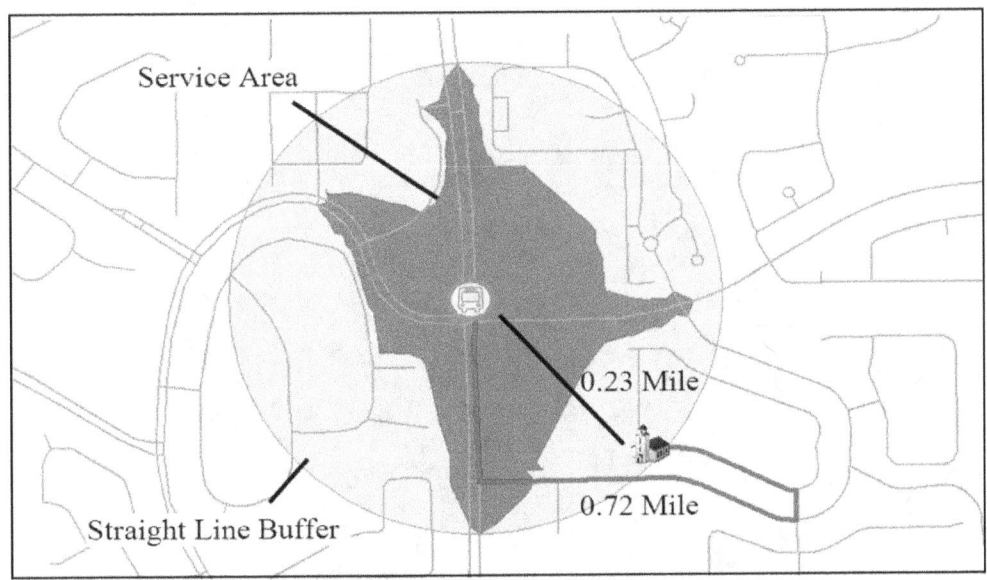

Figure 4-5 Straight-Line Buffer and Service Area.

With ArcGIS Network Analyst, the service areas around any location will be built on a region that encompasses all accessible streets (that is, streets that are within specified impedance) called a network service area. For instance, the five-minute service area for a given point includes all the streets that can be reached within five minutes from that point. In this study, the base street network layer (Figure 4-6) was extracted from the 2005 Tele Atlas.

Because all freeway and ramps prohibit pedestrian use, all freeway and ramps were removed from the street network layer to prevent an incorrectly calculated service area. Figures 4-7 and 4-8 clearly show the difference in the service area with and without the freeway. Figure 4-9 shows all Broward County bus stop service areas based on a quarter-mile straight-line walking distance.

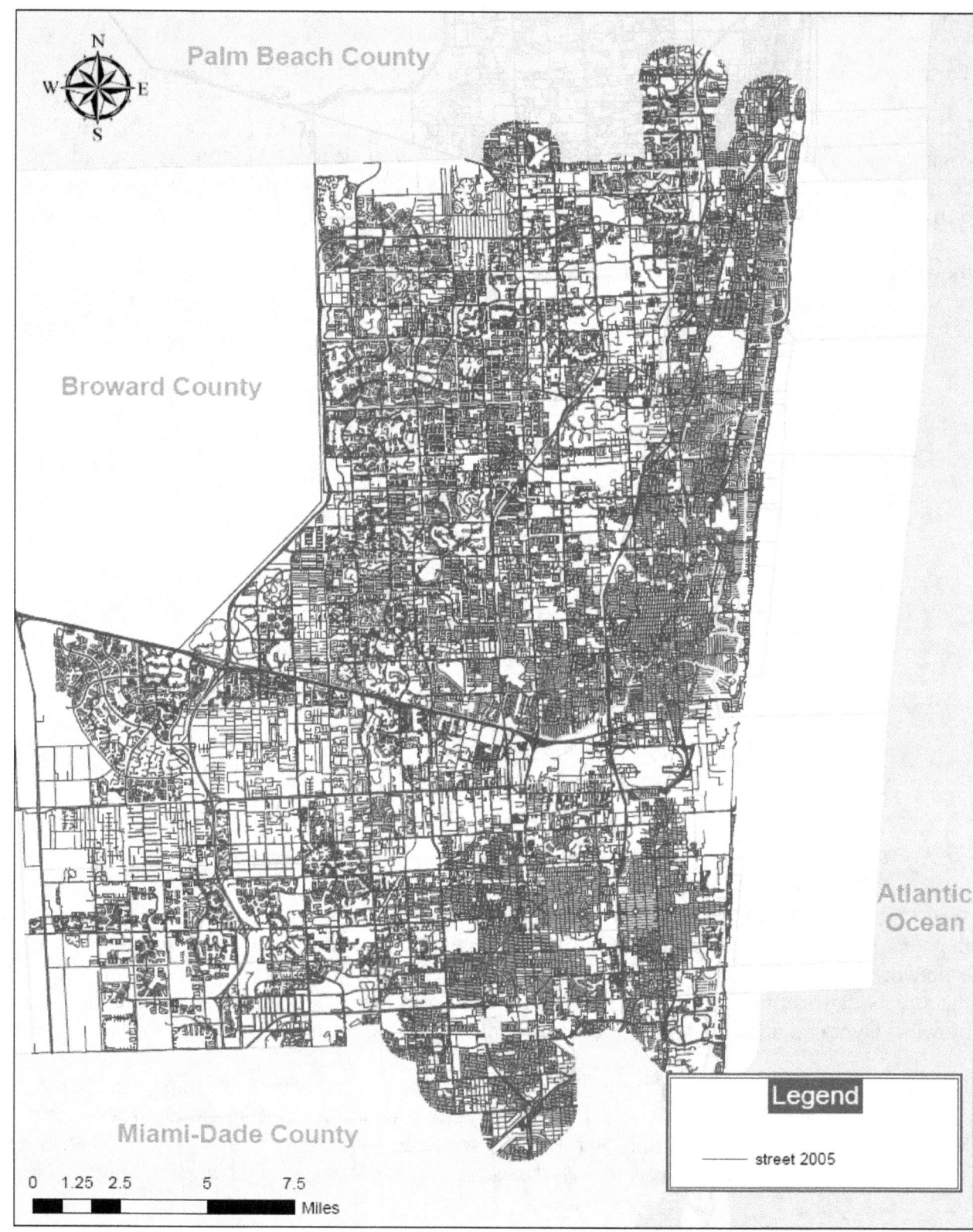

Figure 4-6 Street Network Layer of Broward County.

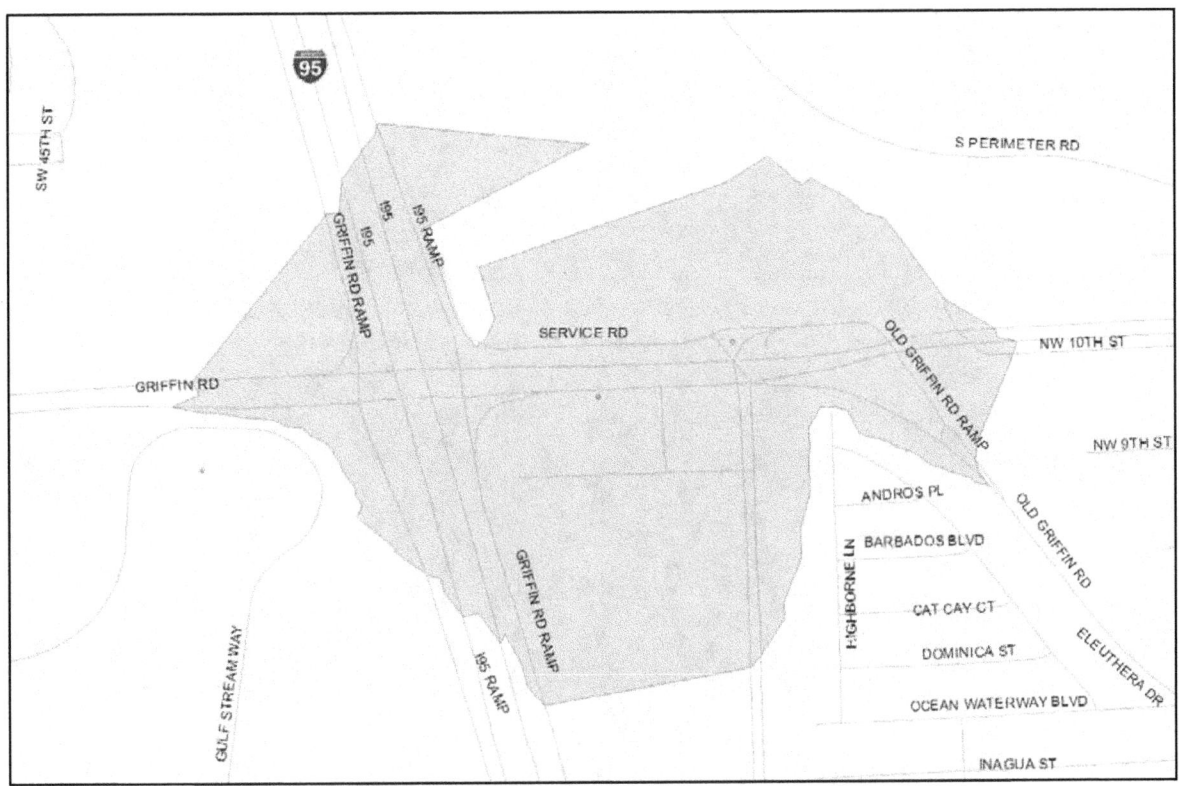

Figure 4-7 Service Area with the Freeway.

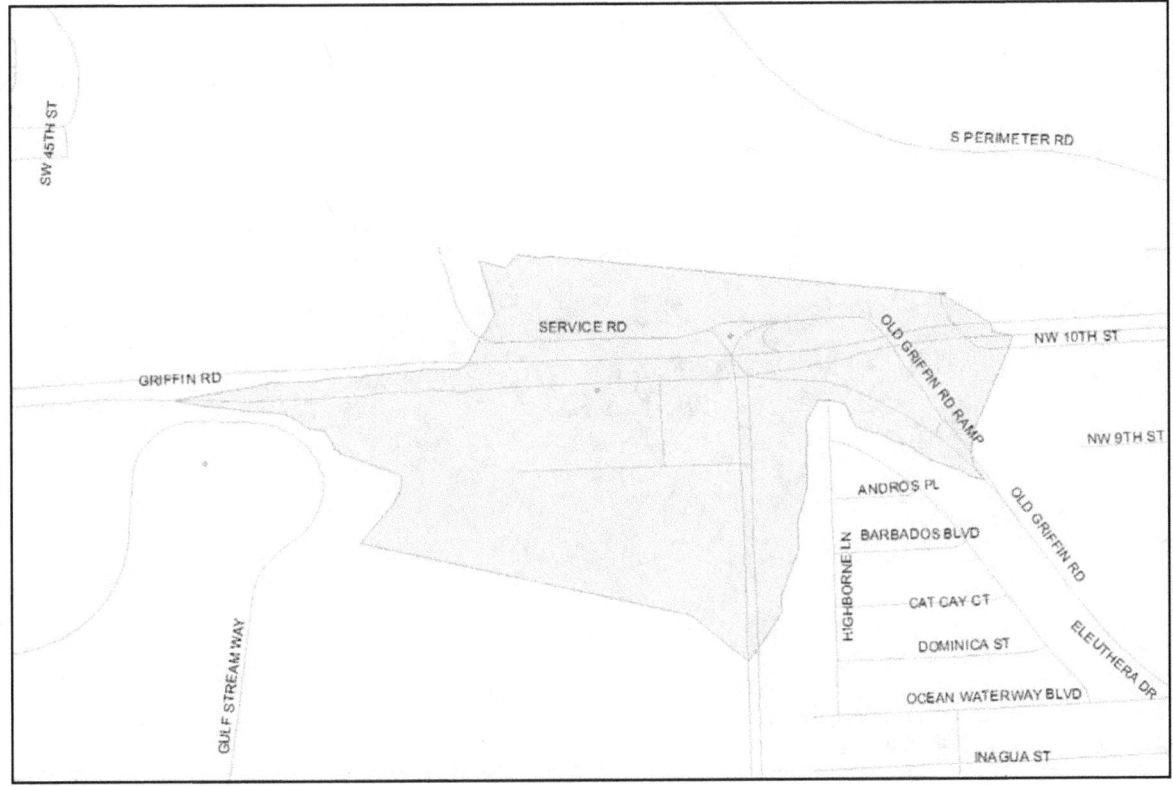

Figure 4-8 Service Area without the Freeway.

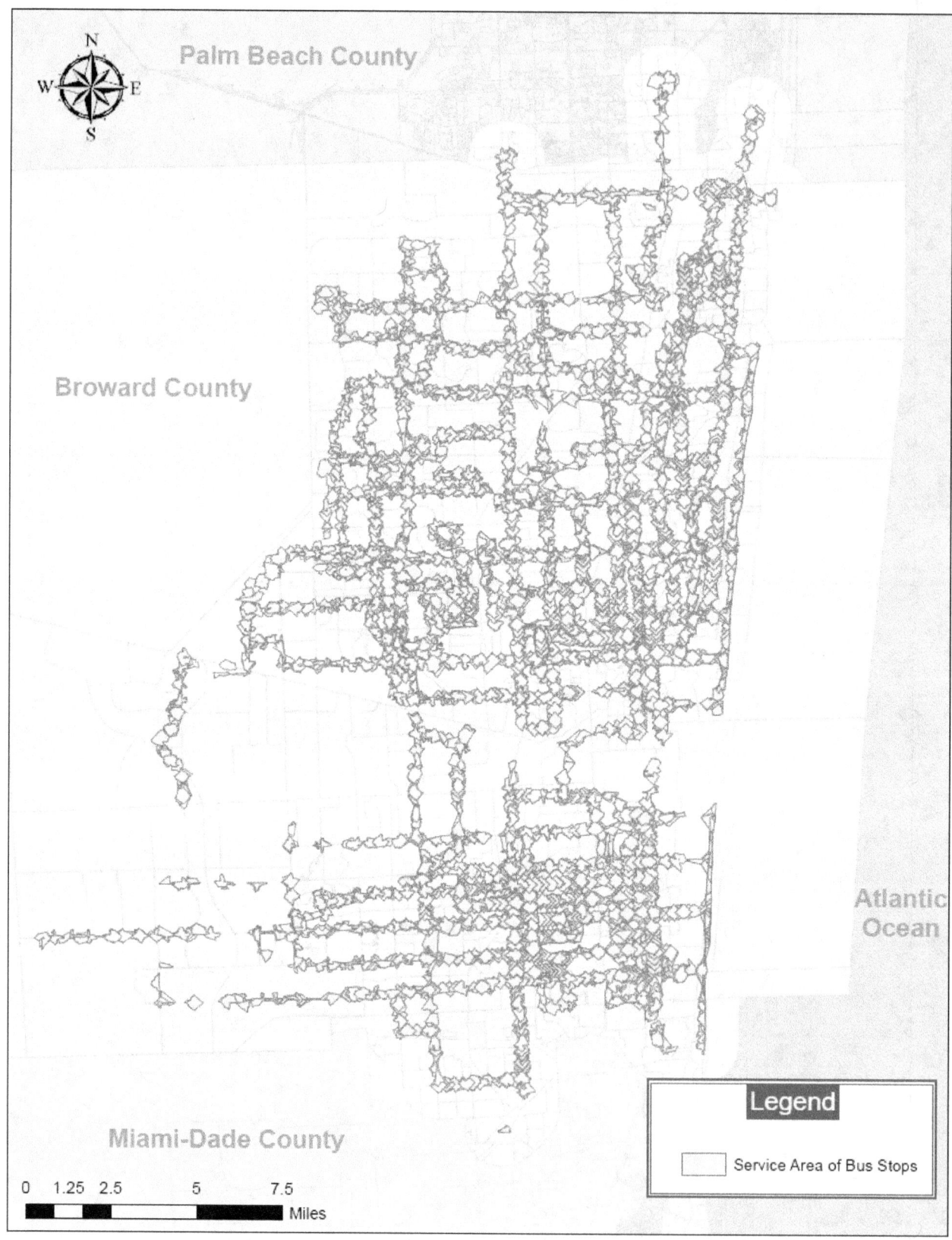

Figure 4-9 Bus Stop Service Area of Broward County.

4.4. Topology of Street Layer

The street network was built from the Tele Atlas street files. Although the Tele Atlas map provides a full and detailed street layer for Broward County, two problems were encountered. The first involved duplicated streets. For example, the selected line in Figure 4-10 has three different records. Second, the selected line in Figure 4-10 represents only a portion of the total walking distance between two intersections, which is usually used to calculate the ADA sidewalk construction improvement. The sidewalk distance, as calculated by the program, requires an integrated single line. Overlapping and incomplete lines will result in integrity and logic problems that will prevent the program from calculating the shortest distance from the bus stop to different facilities on the network.

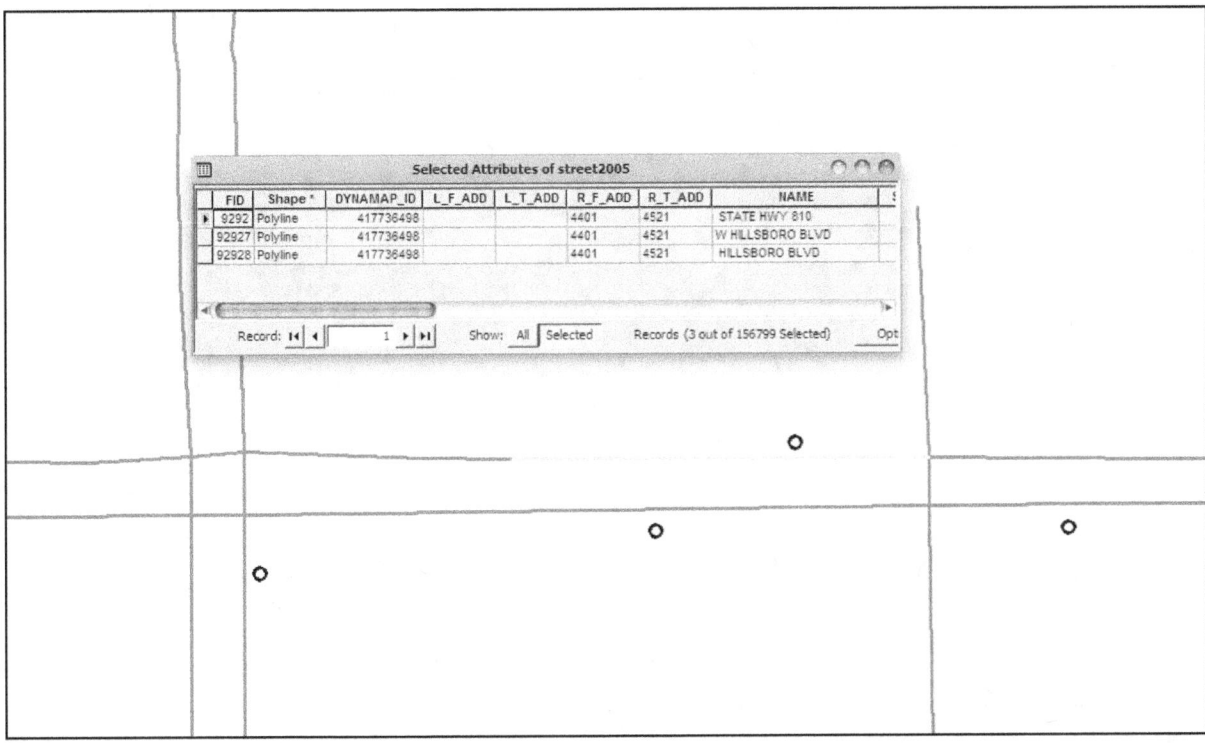

Figure 4-10 Street Layer with Duplicated Record.

The topology function integrated in ArcGIS was applied to solve the problems. Topology has long been a key GIS requirement for data management and integrity. In general, a topological data model represents spatial objects (i.e., point, line, and area features) as an underlying graph of topological primitives—nodes, faces, and edges. These primitives, together with their relationships to one another and to the features whose boundaries they represent, are defined by representing the feature geometries in a planar graph of topological elements. Figures 4-11 and 4-12 show the rules necessary to check and fix overlapping and incomplete lines. The rule "Must Not Overlap" validate that each line in one layer does not overlap lines in the same layer. As indicated in Figure 4-12, the "Must Not Have Pseudos" rule is to check if a line from one layer touches more than one line from the same layer at its endpoints; otherwise, it results in an error message. Figure 4-13 shows the final street layer output.

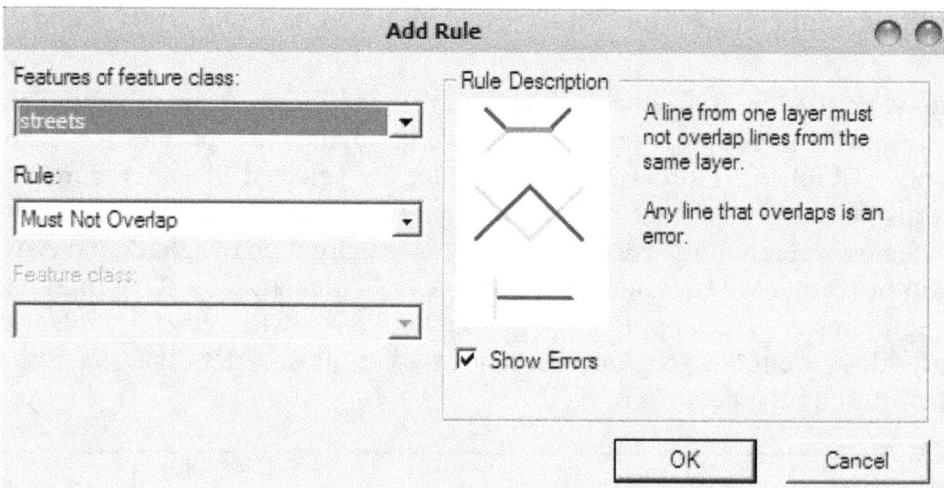

Figure 4-11 Topology Rule "Must Not Overlap".

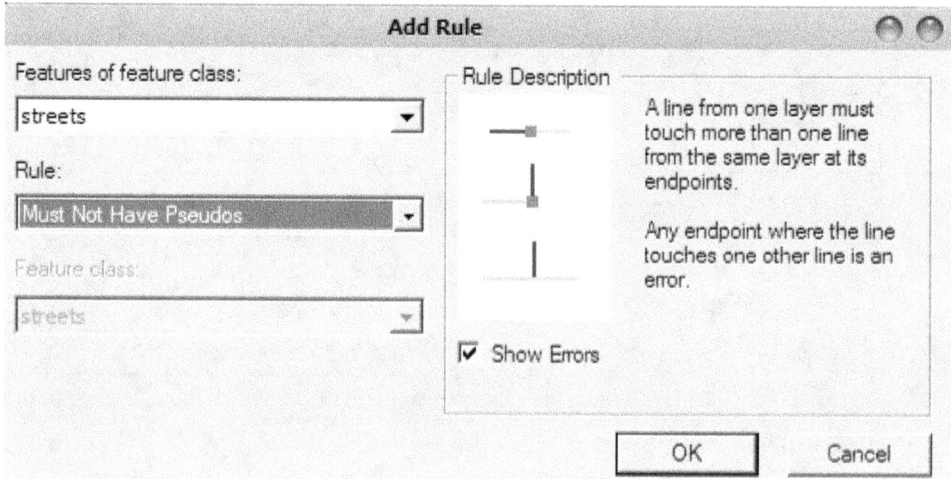

Figure 4-12 Topology Rule "Must Not Have Pseudos".

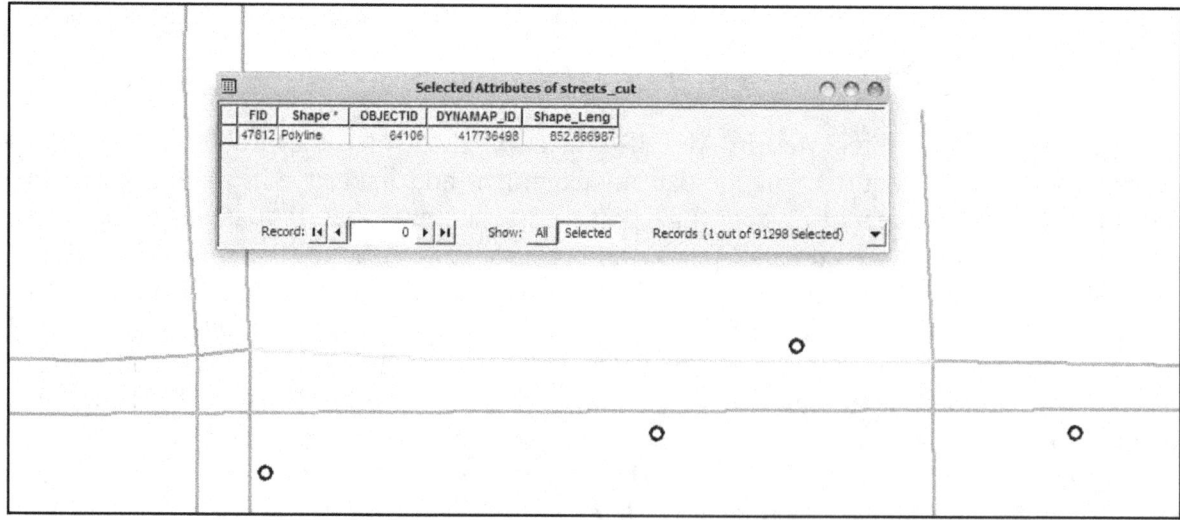

Figure 4-13 Street Layer after Topology Test.

4.5. Score Calculation for Point Layer

One way to evaluate the importance of a service area is the number of facilities it covers. A concentration of facilities and community amenities within the service area of a given bus stop indicates a potentially higher ridership at that bus stop. As mentioned in Subsection 2.4.3, a facility may be located in the overlapping service area of adjacent bus stops. Theoretically, bus riders can choose any one of those bus stops to reach the facility. The probability of choosing the bus stop basically depends on the walking distance to each station. The bus stop nearest to the facility is generally the best choice even if the facility is located in the service area of another bus stop. Counting only the number of facilities within the bus stop service areas would not provide an accurate estimate of the importance score.

As an example, Figure 4-14 shows that two closed bus stops on the same bus route have an overlapping service area. A church is located in the overlapping part of the two separate bus service areas, indicating that buses servicing either stop will reach this church. Counting the number of facilities within the bus stop service areas (the traditional method), this church gets the same weight for each bus stop service area. In reality, the church is closest to the bus stop on the left (0.06 miles walking distance), while the distance to the bus stop on the right is farther (0.20 miles walking distance). Based on common sense, most bus riders would choose the closest stop; this church therefore should have a different weight for each of these two bus stops.

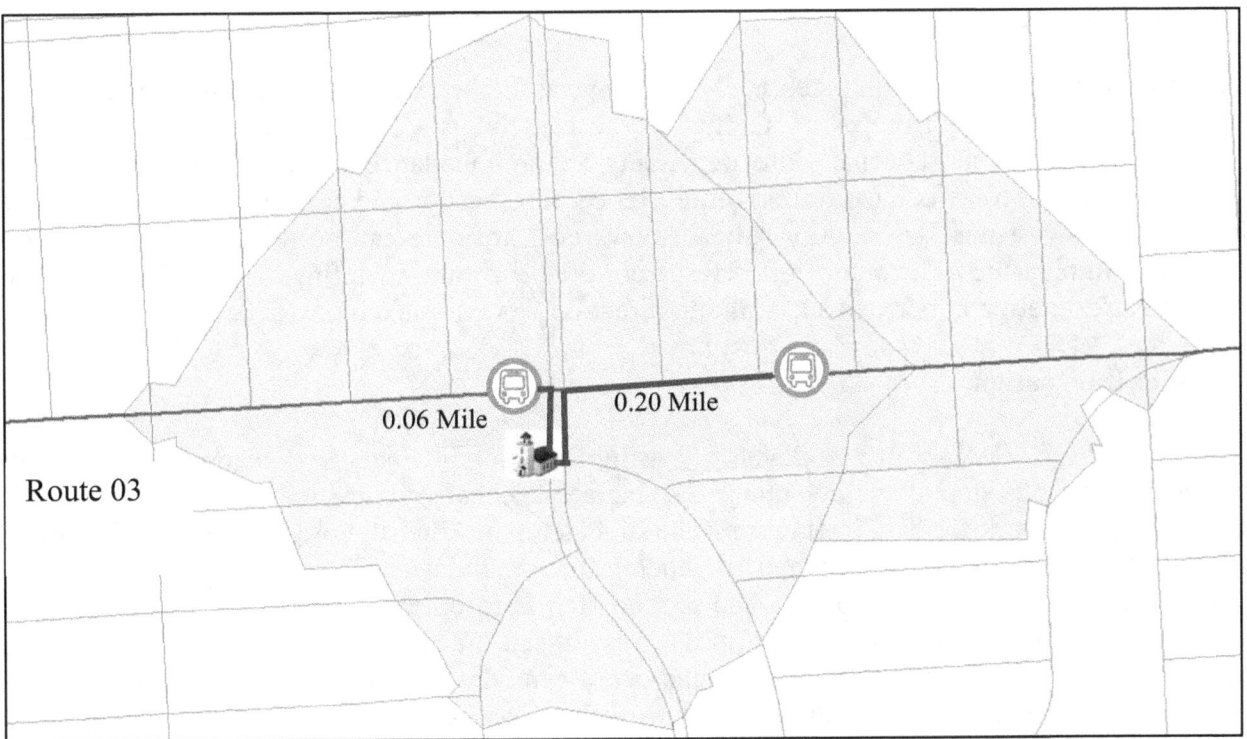

Figure 4-14 Walking Distance in Overlapping Service Area.

A score (s) is used to evaluate the weight of each facility within a bus stop service area based on the equation below:

$$s_{ij} = i_j \cdot p_{ij}$$ (4-1)

where

s_{ij} = the score of the facility j to the bus stop i,

i_j = the importance factor of the facility j,

$p_{ij} = \dfrac{e^{(2-15 \cdot d_{ij})}}{1 + e^{(2-15 d_{ij})}}$, the probability of demand, and

d_{ij} = the shortest walking distance from bus stop i to the facility j.

The score is equal to the importance factor of the facility times the probability weight that riders would walk from the bus stop to the facility. It reflects the ability of the facility to attract traffic volume and simultaneously indicates how easy it is to access the facility from the bus stop. The distance decay function factor for people with disabilities is not available; therefore, Equation 4-1 uses the default numbers of 2 and 15 for intercept parameter a and slope parameter b.

Because ArcGIS Network Analyst is able to perform multiple closest facility analyses simultaneously, it is used to calculate the shortest distance from every facility to the bus stop within the service area. ArcGIS Network Analyst is a powerful extension that provides network-based spatial analysis including routing, travel directions, closest facility, and service area analysis. ArcGIS Network Analyst enables users to dynamically model realistic network conditions, including turn restrictions, speed limits, height restrictions, and traffic conditions, at different times of the day.

As Figure 4-15 shows, the first step is to locate every facility within the service area and then calculate the best route from every facility to the center bus stop. The best route can be the quickest, shortest, or most scenic route, depending on the impedance chosen. If the impedance is time, then the best route is the quickest route. Hence, the "best" route can be defined as the route that has the lowest impedance. Any valid network cost attribute can be used as the impedance when determining the best route. In this research, the best route is defined as the shortest route based on street network; barriers and walking direction were not taken into account.

4.6. Data Integration

In this process, a VBA script was developed using ESRI's ArcObjects extension to integrate all the factors into bus stop status inventory. Service area zones were created as well. Figure 4-16 shows the framework for data integration. The first step is to filter the original bus stop database with ADA accessibility standards and to generate the candidate bus stop database reflecting a need for accessibility improvements. The second step is to combine wheelchair boardings and ridership data into the candidate bus stop database based on bus stop IDs. The third step is to create a quarter-mile service area zone around every candidate bus stop and to integrate the data regarding the population with disabilities, workflow, parks, health care facilities, religious centers, shopping centers, and private and public schools within each buffer zone.

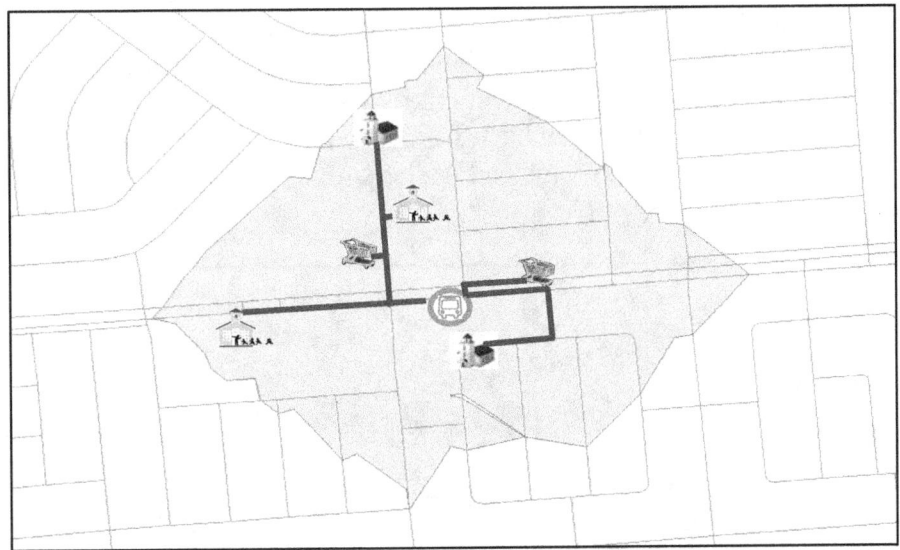

Figure 4-15 Shortest Walking Distance in Service Area.

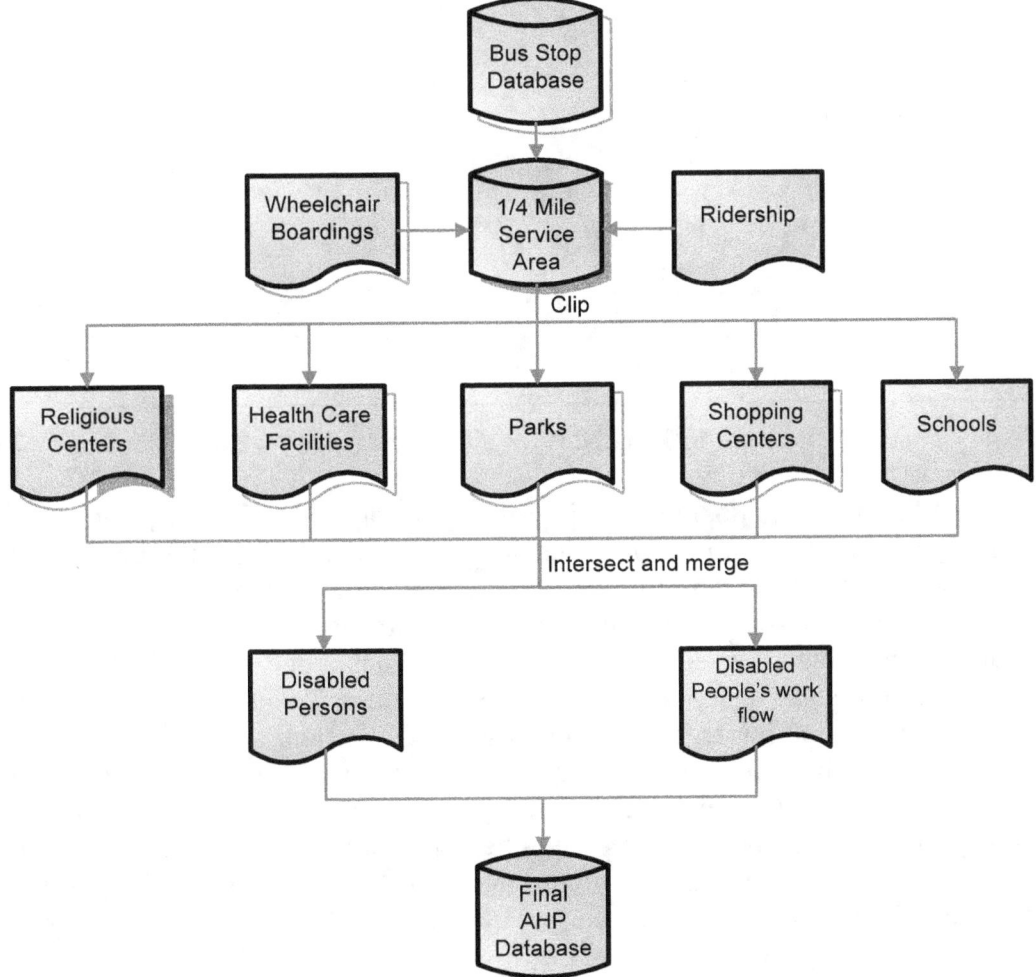

Figure 4-16 Data Integration Framework.

As shown in Figure 4-17, because parks, health care facilities, religious centers, shopping centers, and private and public schools are point data, all the facilities out of the service area boundary will be removed through the "clip" function in ArcGIS. The score S (importance factor times the probability that riders will disembark from a particular bus stop) is used to reflect the weight for ADA bus stop improvements instead of the simple sum of the number for each of the nearby facilities.

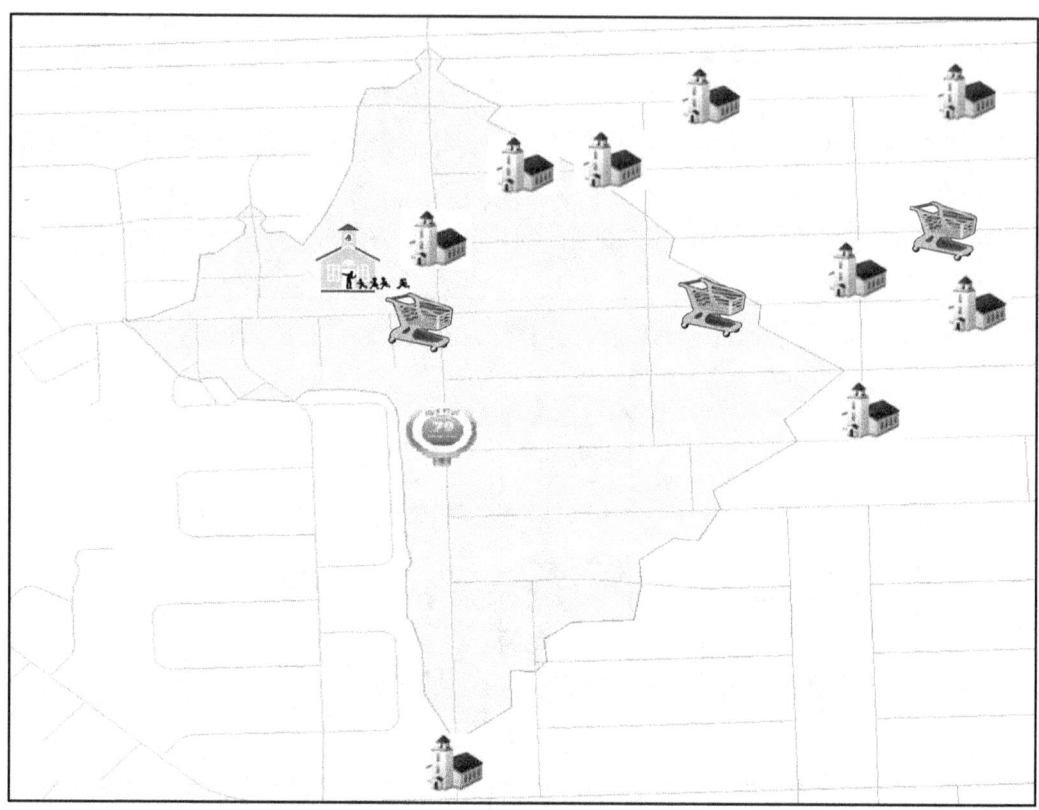

Figure 4-17 Facilities inside the Service Area.

Because the distribution of the population with disabilities and their work trips are both Polygon layers, integrating these data into service area was more complicated. Figure 4-18 shows the integration of five census group zones of the population with disabilities within the center service area. The number in each zone is the number of individuals with disabilities. The first step assumes that this population is evenly distributed in each zone and population density is calculated as such. The second step uses the "intersect" function in ArcGIS to disaggregate the five census group zones and reintegrate them as five small sections within the service area. The final step is to calculate the number of persons with disabilities within each section of the service area by the population density times the updated section. All five updated section populations were added together and the final population numbers generated in the service area indicates that 39 persons with disabilities live in that service area. A VBA program was written to integrate all 5,034 candidate bus stop service areas, the population with disabilities, and work trips. The output for each of the nine factors is shown in Figures 4-19 to 4-27, respectively. Finally, the scores for all candidate bus stops for all criteria were combined into a single database for use in an analytical hierarchy process (AHP) analysis.

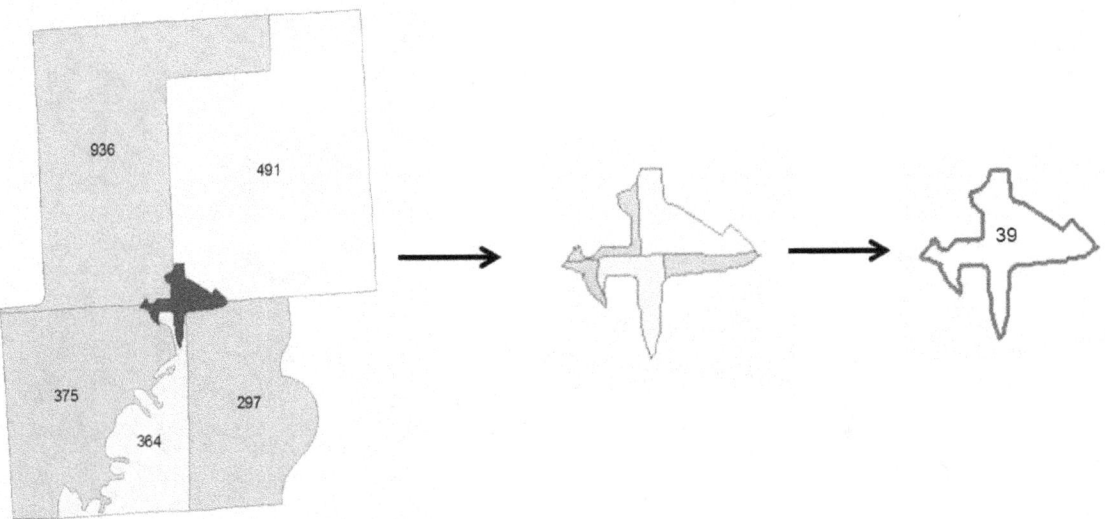

Figure 4-18 Calculate the Population with Disabilities inside the Service Area.

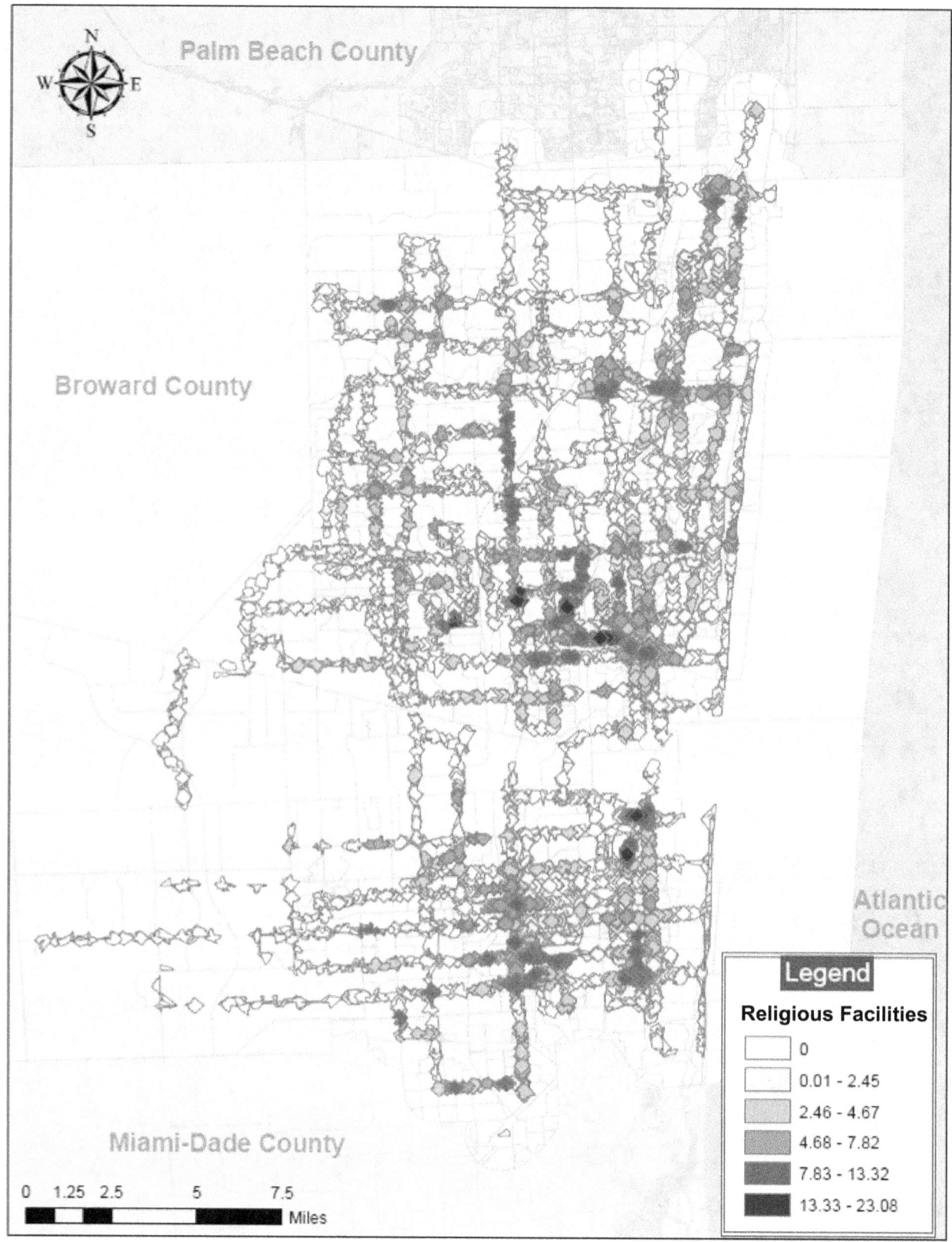

Figure 4-19 Religious Facilities within One Quarter-Mile Service Area of Each Bus Stop.

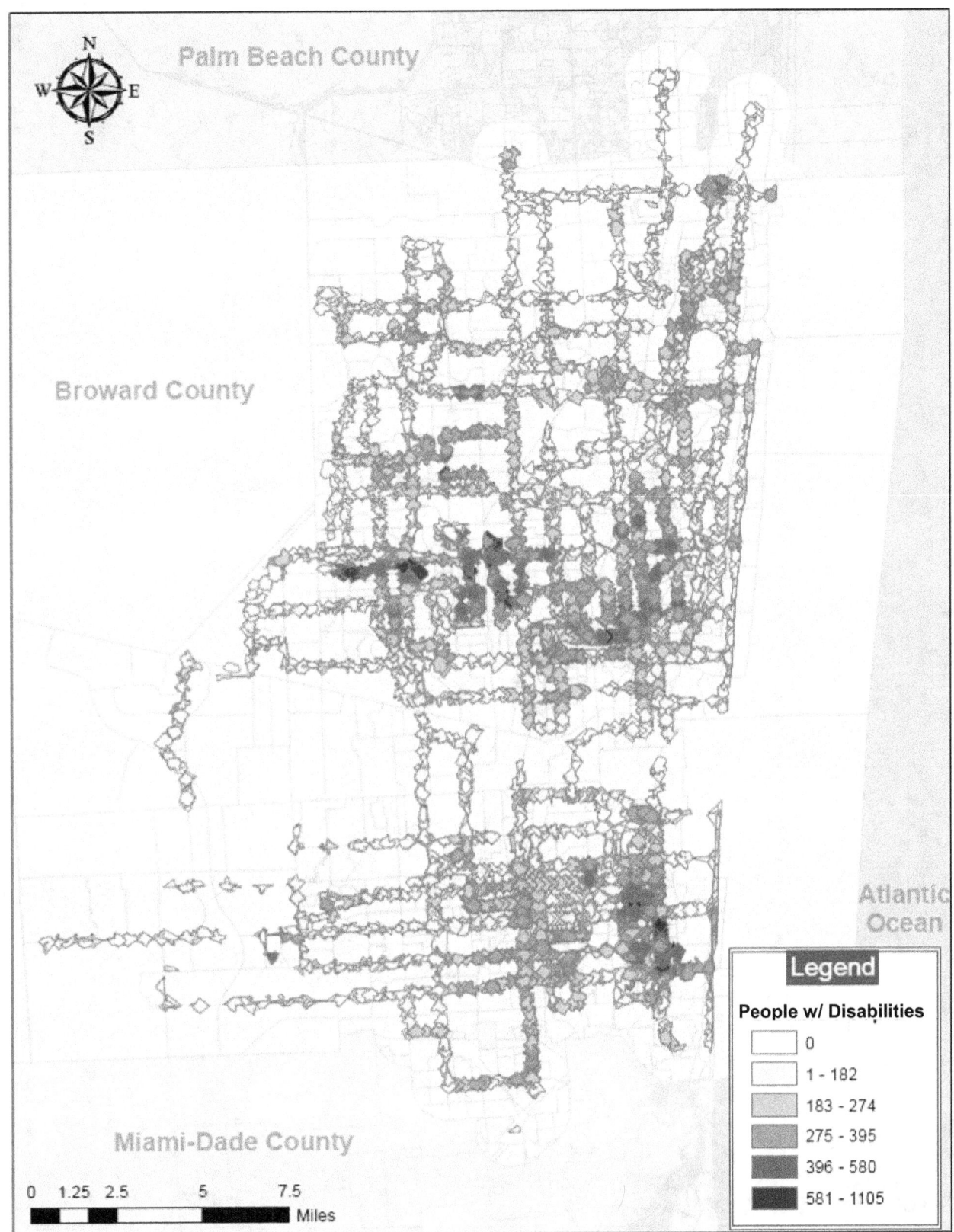

Figure 4-20 People with Disabilities within One Quarter-Mile Service Area of Each Bus Stop.

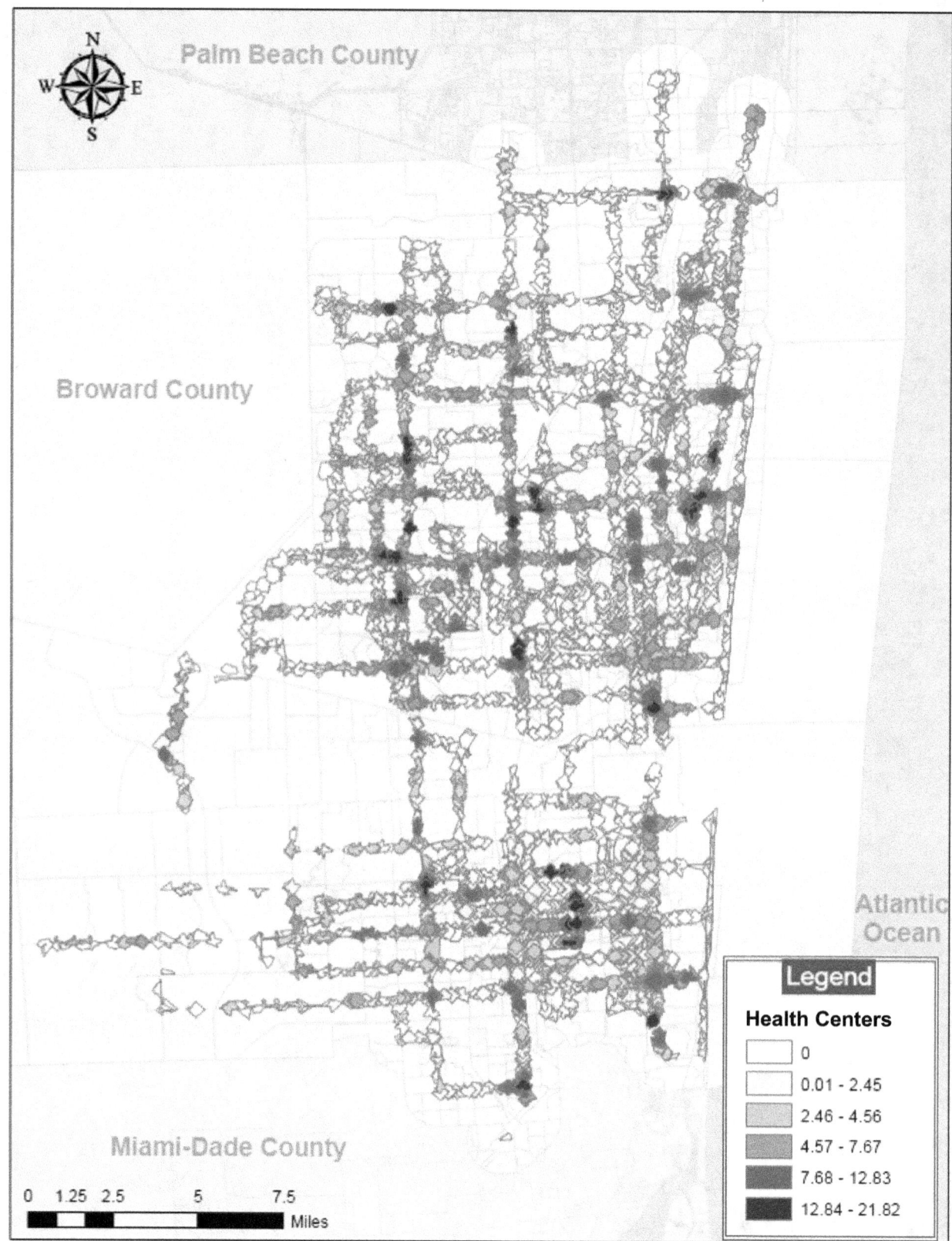

Figure 4-21 Health Centers within the Quarter-Mile Service Area of Each Bus Stop.

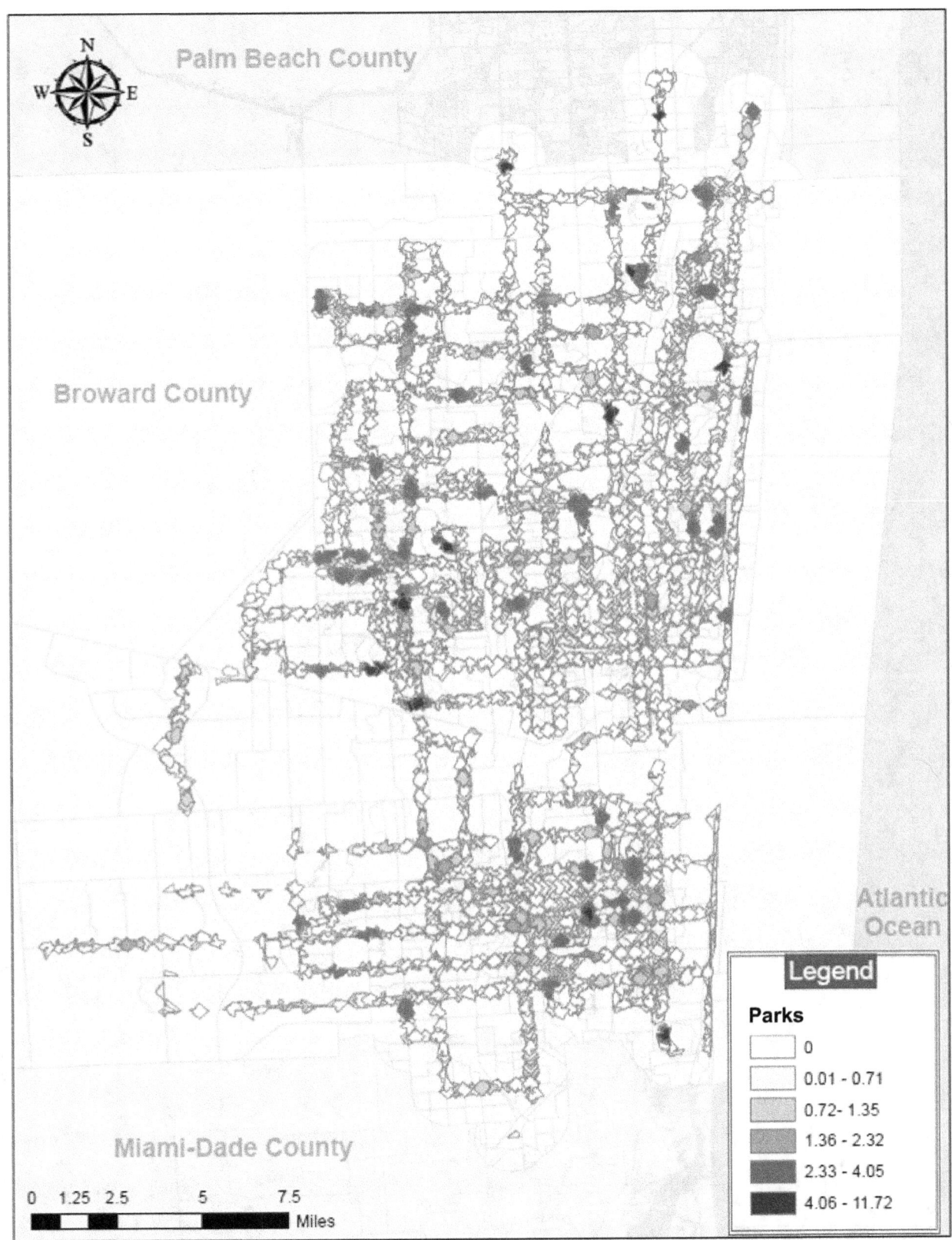

Figure 4-22 Parks within One Quarter-Mile Service Area of Each Bus Stop.

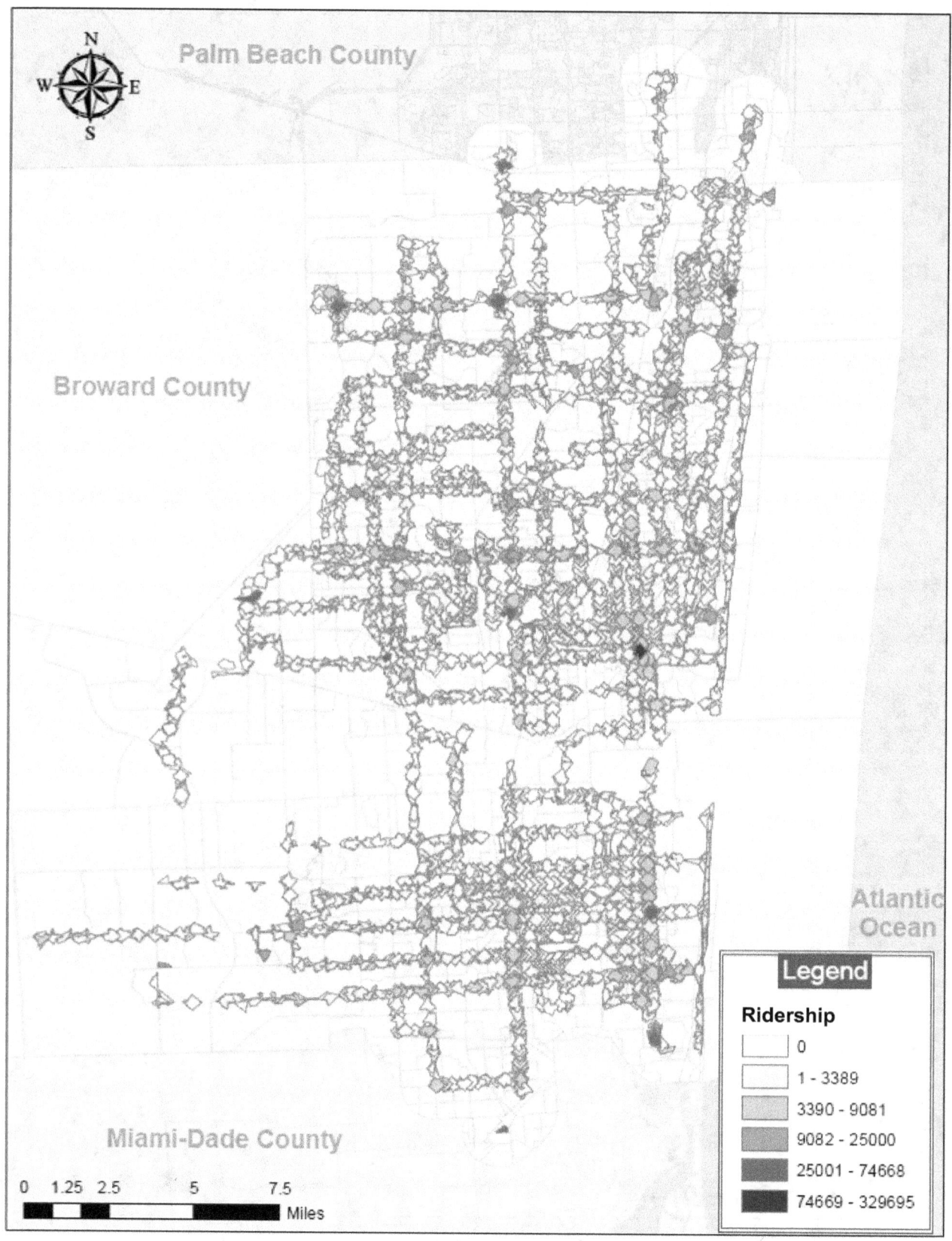

Figure 4-23 Ridership per Bus Stop.

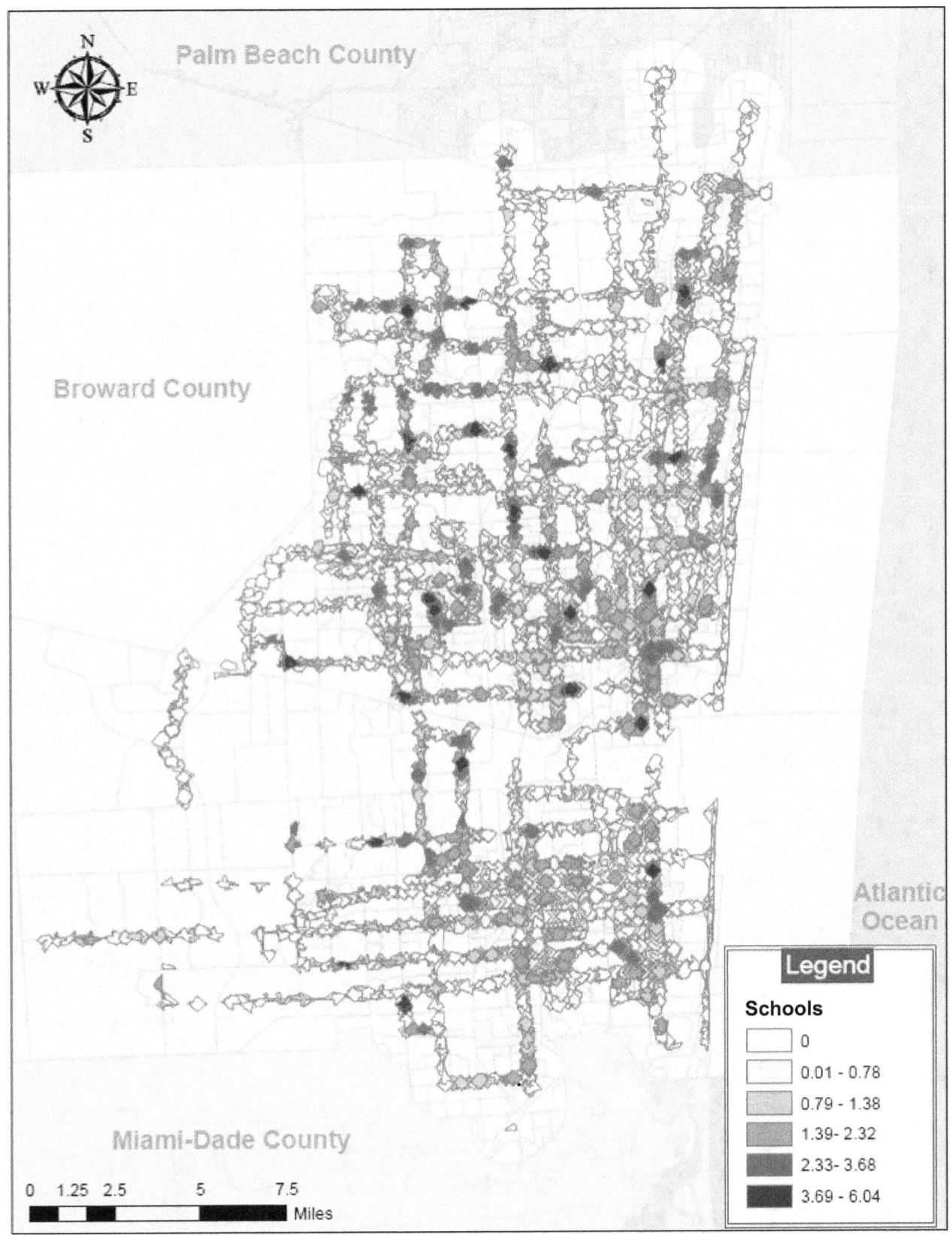

Figure 4-24 Schools within One Quarter-Mile Service Area of Each Bus Stop.

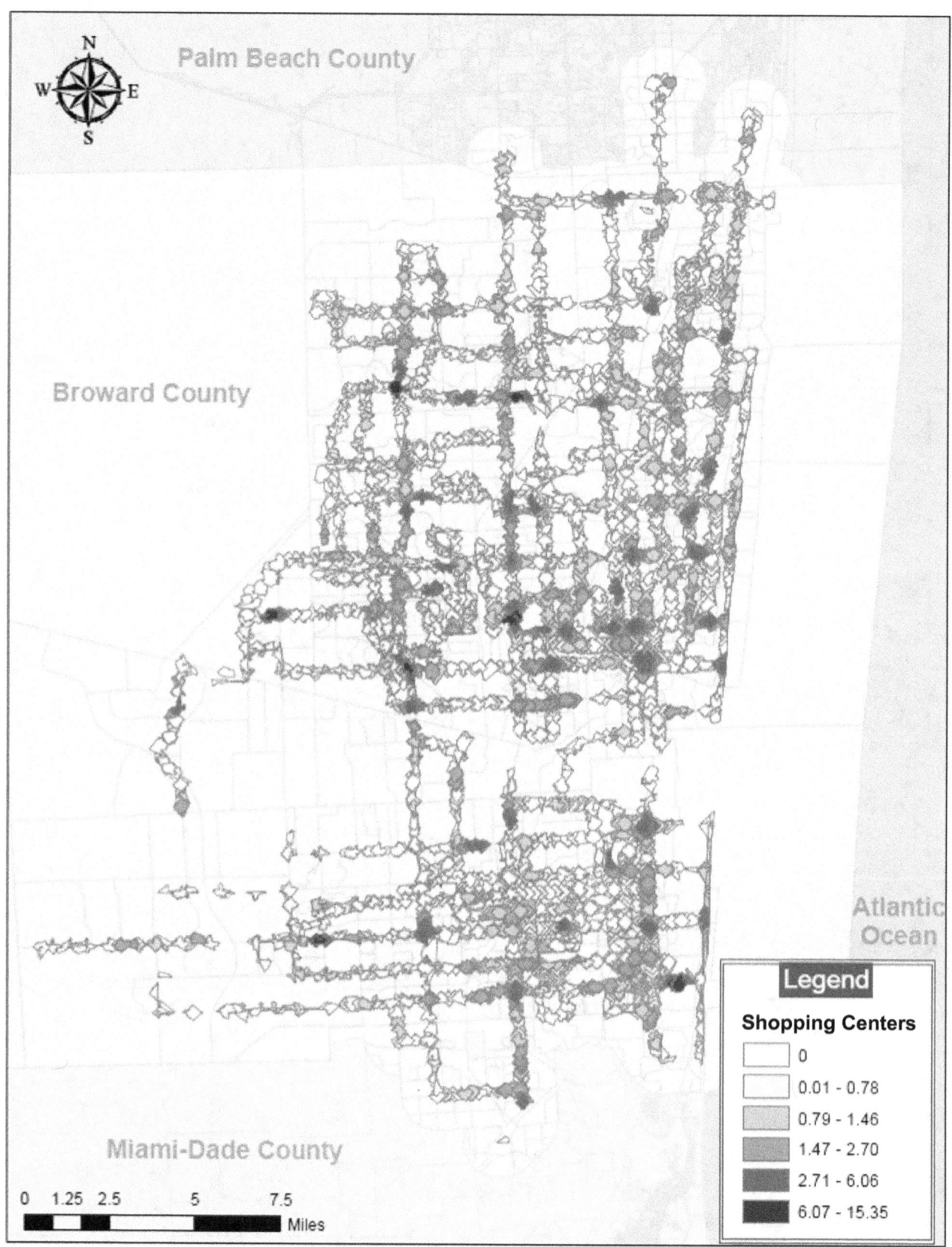

Figure 4-25 Shopping Centers within One Quarter-Mile Service Area of Each Bus Stop.

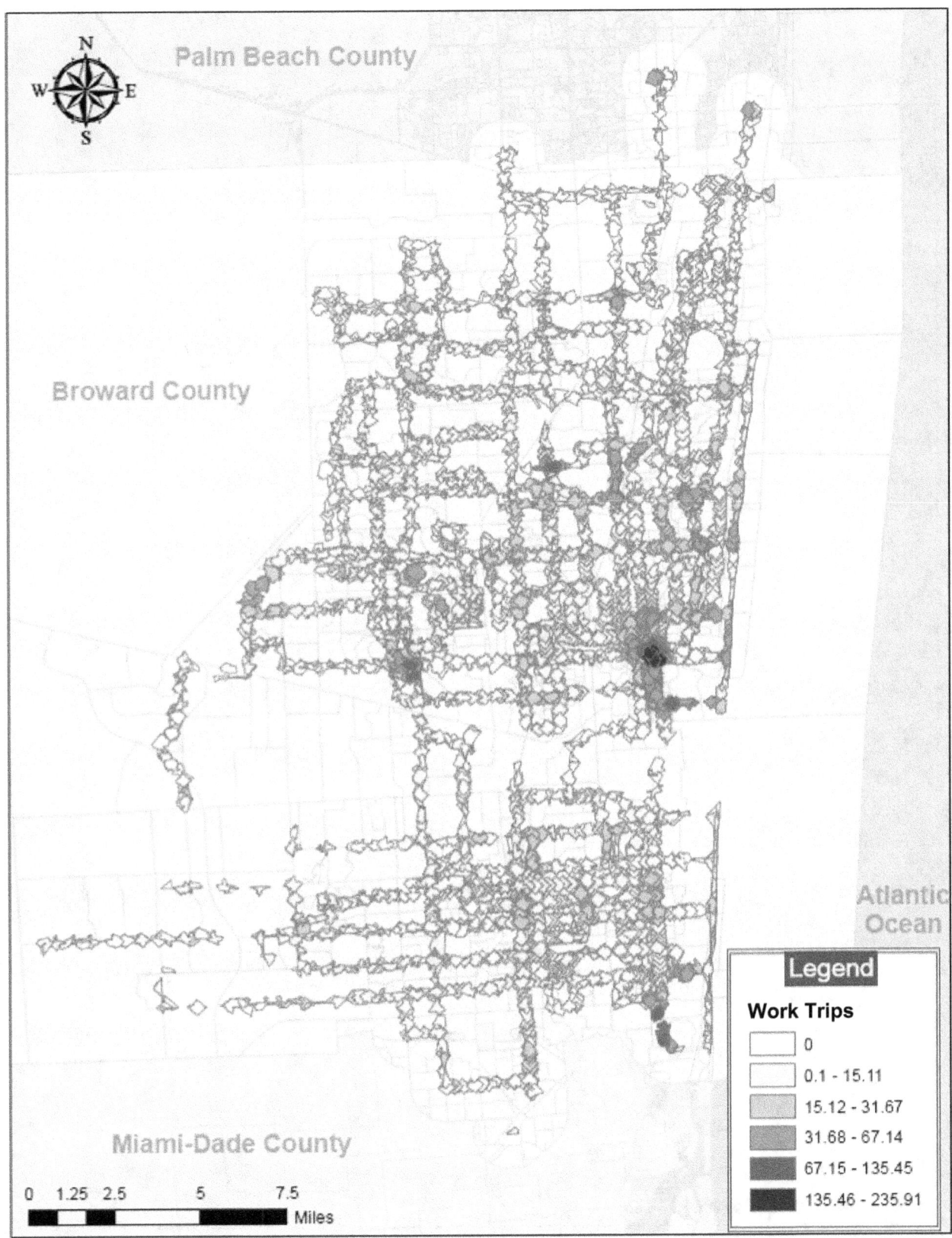

Figure 4-26 Work Trips by Persons with Disabilities within One Quarter-Mile of Each Bus Stop.

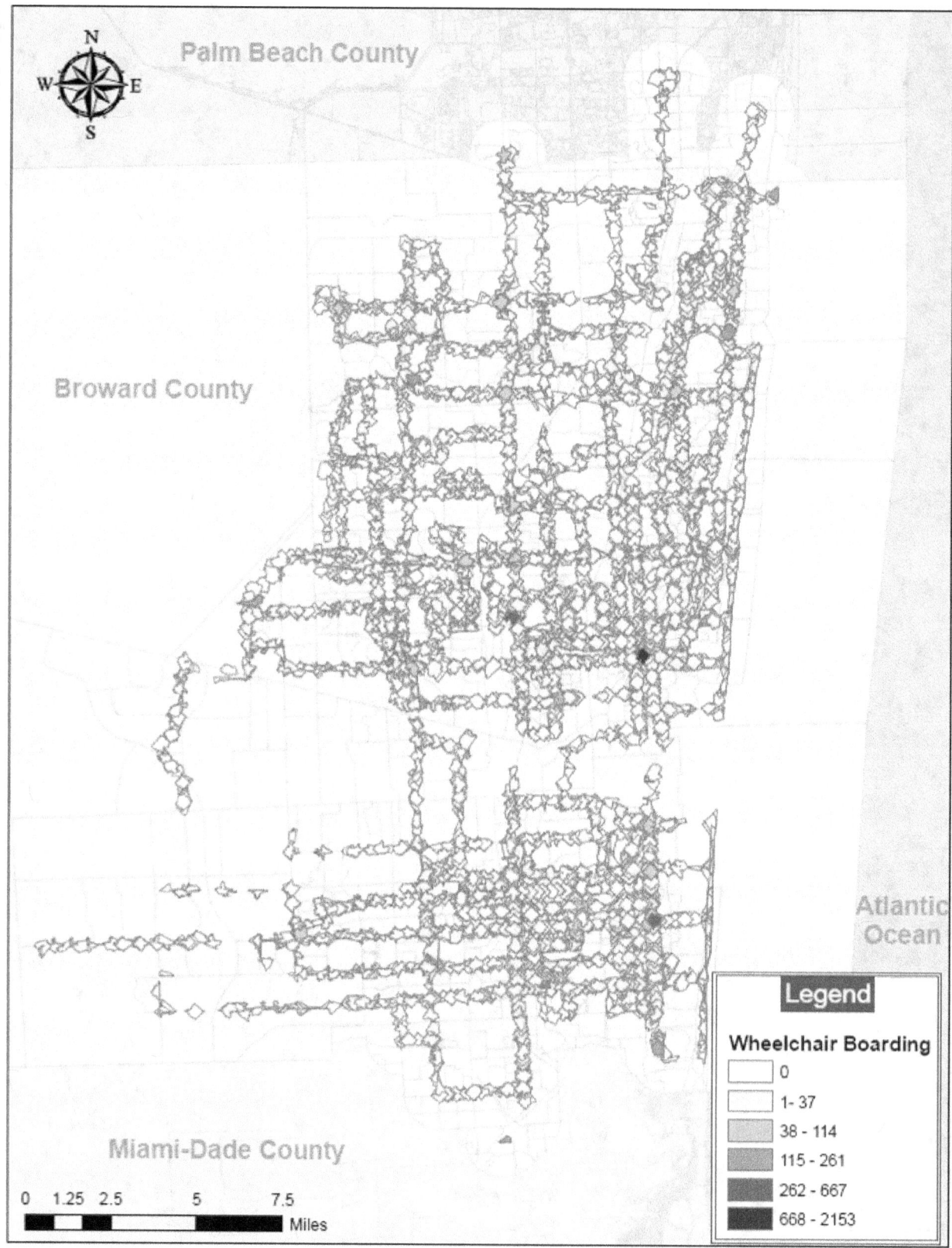

Figure 4-27 Wheelchair Boarding within One Quarter-Mile of Each Bus Stop.

4.7. Correlation Analysis

Nine factors were considered in the AHP process. A correlation analysis was performed to test the correlation among these factors using the equation below:

$$\rho_{XY} = \frac{\text{cov}(X,Y)}{\sqrt{Var(X) \cdot Var(Y)}} \tag{4-2}$$

where

ρ_{XY} = the correlation coefficient between two random variables X and Y,
$cov(X,Y)$ = the covariance of two dataset X and Y,
$Var(X)$ = the variance of X, and
$Var(Y)$ = the variance of X.

Table 4-7 provides all the correlation coefficients. It shows that most factors have a lower correlation coefficient between each other; the relationship between ridership and wheelchair boardings, however, has the highest correlation coefficient 0.9416. This correlation coefficient is higher because wheelchair boardings can be treated as a subclass of overall ridership data; wheelchair boardings are higher as general ridership increases, especially at interchange bus stops. In addition, wheelchair boardings and ridership data were all collected from the same data source through automatic passenger counters (APCs). Due to the limited nature of the wheelchair boarding data (in large part, bus stops did not have wheelchair boarding data), and the higher correlation with the ridership data, general ridership can reflect the importance of the stop to persons in wheelchairs. Ultimately, the "wheelchair boarding" factor was removed and the remaining eight factors were loaded into AHP.

Table 4-7 Correlations Coefficients of the Nine Original Criteria.

ρ_{XY}	Church	Health Center	Park	School	Shop	Persons with Disabilities	Work Trips	Rider-ship	Wheel-chair Boardings
Church	1.0000	0.1100	-0.0310	0.1699	0.1528	0.2343	0.0575	0.0341	0.0292
Health Center	0.1100	1.0000	0.0593	0.0971	0.2058	0.0308	0.1433	0.0412	0.0199
Park	-0.0310	0.0593	1.0000	-0.0074	-0.0084	0.0026	-0.0098	0.0068	-0.0067
School	0.1699	0.0971	-0.0074	1.0000	0.0723	0.0427	0.1328	0.0202	0.0140
Shop	0.1528	0.2058	-0.0084	0.0723	1.0000	0.0558	0.1886	0.1286	0.1213
Persons with Disabilities	0.2343	0.0308	0.0026	0.0427	0.0558	1.0000	0.0350	0.0141	0.0141
Work trips	0.0575	0.1433	-0.0098	0.1328	0.1886	0.0350	1.0000	0.1379	0.1191
Ridership	0.0341	0.0412	0.0068	0.0202	0.1286	0.0141	0.1379	1.0000	0.9416
Wheelchair Boardings	0.0292	0.0199	-0.0067	0.0140	0.1213	0.0141	0.1191	0.9416	1.0000

4.8. Analytic Hierarchy Process (AHP)

As mentioned, AHP is a multicriteria decision-making (MCDM) technique that can combine qualitative and quantitative factors for prioritizing, ranking, and evaluating alternatives (Moldovanyi, 2004). In this research, AHP was used to compare and evaluate the different criteria within every candidate bus stop service area. A total of eight criteria were considered, each assigned a specified weight, based on: 1) the distribution of the population with disabilities; 2) bus ridership per bus stop; 3) transportation to work data for persons with disabilities; and 4) the number of health care facilities, hospitals, parks, religious centers, schools, and shopping centers located within a specified distance from the bus stop in question. AHP consists of three stages described below.

4.8.1. Standardizing the Criteria

The raw score of each criterion for each candidate bus stop was first standardized using the equation below:

$$x'_{ij} = \frac{x_{ij}}{x_j^{max}}$$

(4-3)

where

x'_{ij} = the standardized score for candidate bus stop i for criterion j,

x_j^{max} = the maximum score for criterion j, and

x_{ij} = the raw score for candidate bus stop i for criterion j.

The benchmark score (x_j^{max}) was used to compare the scores among the candidate bus stops. For the minimum ADA improvements, x_j^{max} is the maximum score among the bus stops that did not meet the minimum ADA standards based on criterion j. Similarly, for universal design improvements, x_j^{max} is the maximum score among the bus stops that did not meet the universal standards based on criterion j (e.g., having no shelter or bench).

4.8.2. Weighting Standardized Criteria

The AHP uses composite weights to represent ratings of alternatives with respect to an overall goal. The weights, also referred to as decision alternatives scores, are the basis for making decisions. They serve to rate the effectiveness of each alternative in achieving the goal. The overall score for a candidate bus stop is defined as follows:

$$R_i = \sum_j w_j x'_{ij}$$

(4-4)

where

R_i = the overall score of candidate bus stop i, and

w_j = the vector of priorities associated with criterion j, $\sum w_j = 1$.

Note that the weight, w_j, is an important factor in AHP. It requires assessing the relative importance of different criteria, understanding that different assigned weights will result in different output selections. Hence, an experienced decision maker or senior transit planner usually assigns weights. By comparison and analysis, the travel patterns and percentage of riders with disabilities derived in Table 2-2 informed the default weights used for each criterion shown in Table 4-8 for both minimum ADA and universal design standards. Given that bus stop service areas with higher populations with disabilities necessitate meeting ADA accessibility service requirements directly, residential locations in areas that have a high population of people with disabilities should receive the highest weight. Ridership represents the number of boardings for each bus stop; hence, this number was considered the second-most-important criterion. The locations of religious centers, health care facilities, parks, shopping centers, and schools selected as common destinations for persons with disabilities, were treated with the third highest weight. Because universal design also benefits other bus riders, the weight in universal design was higher than the minimum ADA improvement level.

Table 4-8 Default Weights for Criteria.

Criteria	Weights (w_j) for Minimum ADA Standards	Weights (w_j) for Universal Design Standards
Religious Center Facility	0.035	0.035
Population w/ Disabilities Location	0.300	0.150
Health Care Facilities	0.100	0.100
Parks	0.035	0.035
Private and Public School	0.100	0.100
Shopping Centers	0.080	0.080
Work Trips by Persons with Disabilities	0.150	0.150
Ridership per Stop	0.200	0.350

4.8.3. Standardizing Weighted Criterion

The overall score R_i from the second stage was further standardized using the equation below:

$$R_i' = \frac{R_i}{\sum R_i} \qquad (4\text{-}5)$$

where
R_i'= the standardized overall score of candidate bus stop i, and
R_i = the overall score of candidate bus stop i.

A user-friendly VBA program was developed to perform all the calculations involved in the above three stages. The program produced the final score for each candidate bus stop, which serves as one of the two major inputs to the optimization model to be described below. The other major input, the project budget and construction cost estimates, is detailed in the next chapter. Figures 4-28 and 4-29 show the R_i' value for the minimum ADA and universal design standards respectively.

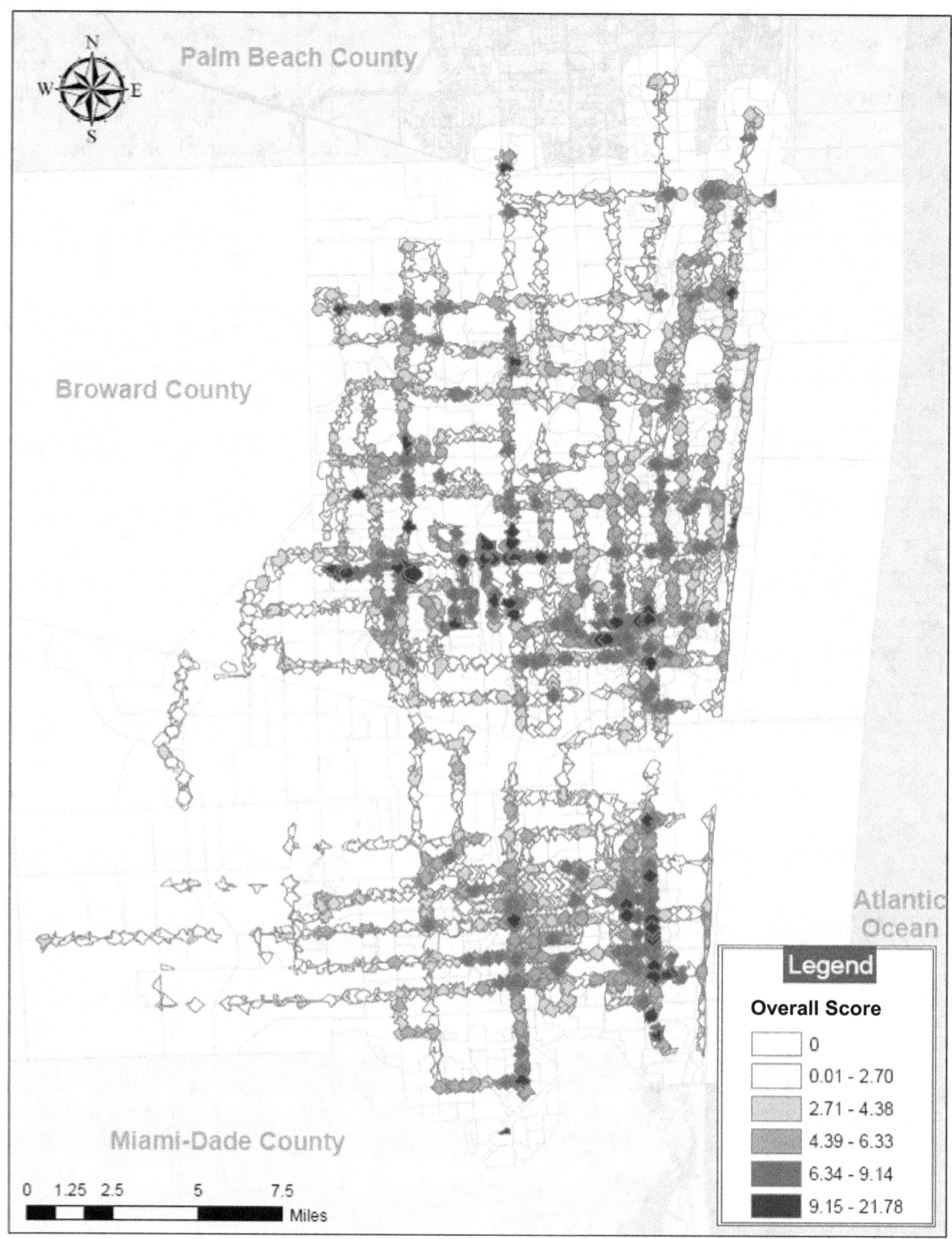

Figure 4-28 Overall Score Based on Minimum ADA Standards.

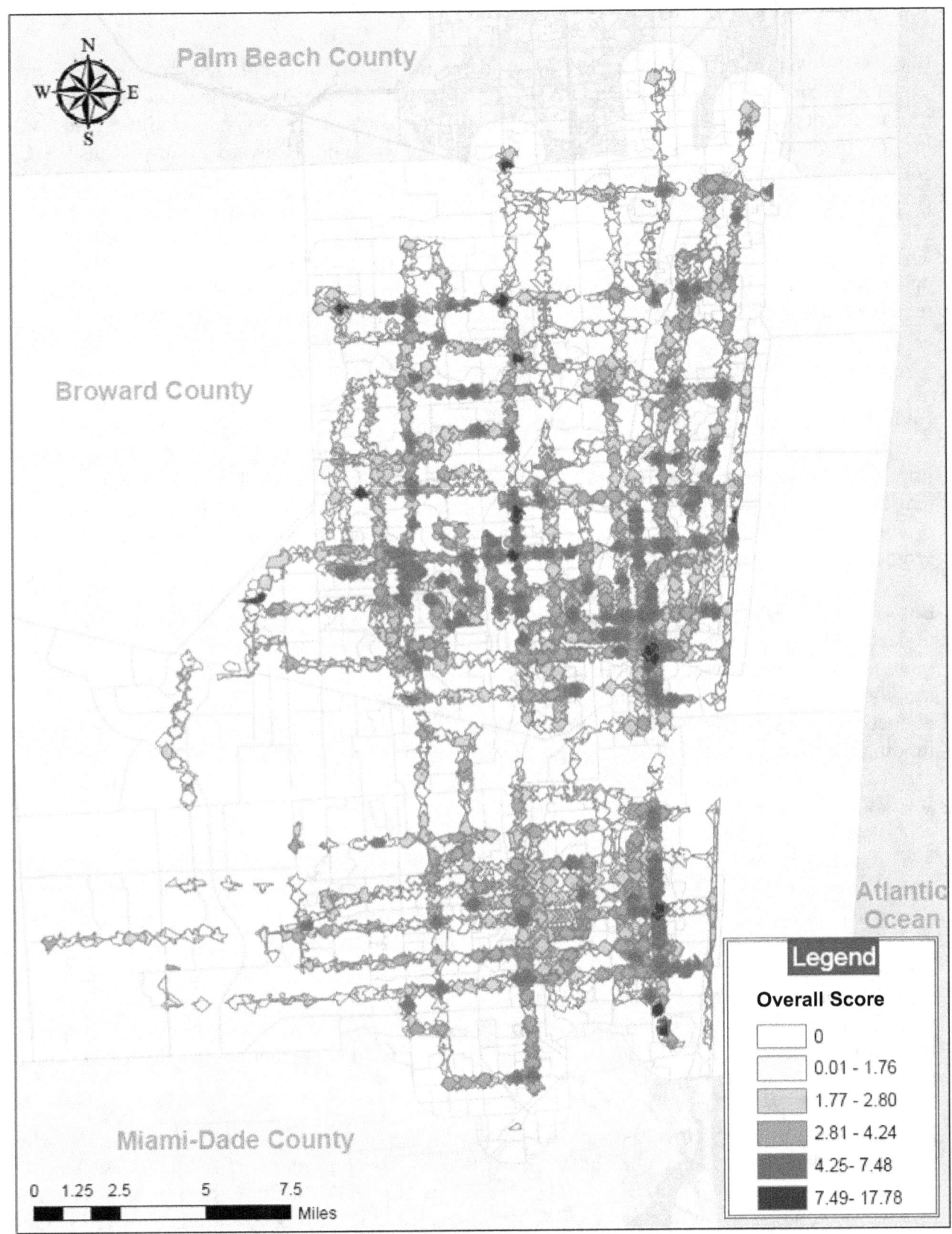

Figure 4-29 Overall Score Based on Universal Design Standards.

4.9. Budget and Cost Estimates

Budget and cost estimates are critical input to the optimization model. The budget is the main constraint that limits the number of bus stops assigned for construction needed to meet ADA improvements each year. The budget also reflects how transit agencies invest in ADA improvements. Cost estimates were collected from the two major Broward County Transit (BCT) contractors. The estimates cover all kinds of costs for bus stop ADA improvements, such as the cost of the design, maintenance of traffic, material, and construction. Based on the cost estimation, a detailed cost list (including the cost to meet the minimum ADA standards and the cost to meet universal design standards) for each candidate bus stop was developed for the optimization model. Considering that some bus stops share the same sidewalks, which will cause redundant calculations, certain stops were filtered as special groups for cost estimation.

4.9.1. Assigned Budget for Transit ADA Improvements

Budgetary information was mainly derived from the Broward County Transit Development Plan (TDP) and the Broward County Metropolitan Planning Organization Transportation Improvement Program (TIP) (Broward County Transit, 2005). The TDP is a short-range plan that addresses operational and capital improvements for BCT; the TIP is a short-range plan produced annually for the allocation of resources over each of the upcoming five-year periods by project phase.

Based on data in the TDP, bus stop ADA improvements belong under the replacement/maintenance program for facilities of the mass transit capital plan. In accordance with the Americans with Disabilities Act (ADA), BCT works to enhance the countywide mobility of persons with disabilities by maximizing accessibility to public transit. The assigned budget for ADA transit improvements is $2.0 million per year from 2006 to 2010. Although funding for shelter and bench improvements came from a different budget, they were counted as part of the total budget for ADA improvements as these facilities are highly related to the accessibility of bus stops for persons with disabilities.

4.9.2. Cost Estimation for Bus Stop ADA Improvements

Cost calculations for ADA bus stop improvements cannot assure that the projected cost will be exactly the same as that for the actual construction work. Construction costs vary with different contractors, and costs with regard to bus stop improvements will likely change during construction due to inflation or other unforeseen factors. This study can only make reasonable cost estimates for each bus stop based on the current two major contractors working with Broward County Transit. Design, traffic maintenance, and construction usually make up the general cost of improvements.

Minimum ADA improvements concentrated on sidewalks, loading pads, and curb cuts, while universal design improvement included shelters, benches, bus maps, and schedules. To meet minimum ADA improvements, the cost estimation for sidewalks, loading pads, and curb cuts are relatively simple. The two fields "CURB_CUT" and "LOAD_PAD" from the Broward County bus stop maintenance database were used to make the decision; "Y" indicates the facility exists and does not need improvement and "N" indicates otherwise.

For sidewalk ADA improvements, the fields "b_SIDEWALK" and "SIDEWALK_W" were used to calculate construction cost. The first field indicates that a sidewalk is present and the second field provides the actual width of the sidewalk. If the width of the sidewalk is less than three feet, the sidewalk needs ADA improvement; although BCT cannot afford to provide ADA-qualified sidewalks from the bus stop to the door of every facility, this information is invaluable in assisting decisions about these improvements at specific sites. Sidewalk length was considered the distance between the two nearest intersections where the bus stops are located, as shown in Figure 4-30. A VBA ArcGIS integrated program calculated the sidewalk length for every candidate bus stop.

The detailed sidewalk ADA improvement cost includes concrete sidewalk construction, concrete curb-and-cutter if there is no existing sidewalk, sidewalk concrete removal if the existing sidewalk does not meet the ADA standards, and subgrade preparation for concrete pour. The detailed unit costs are given in Table 4-9.

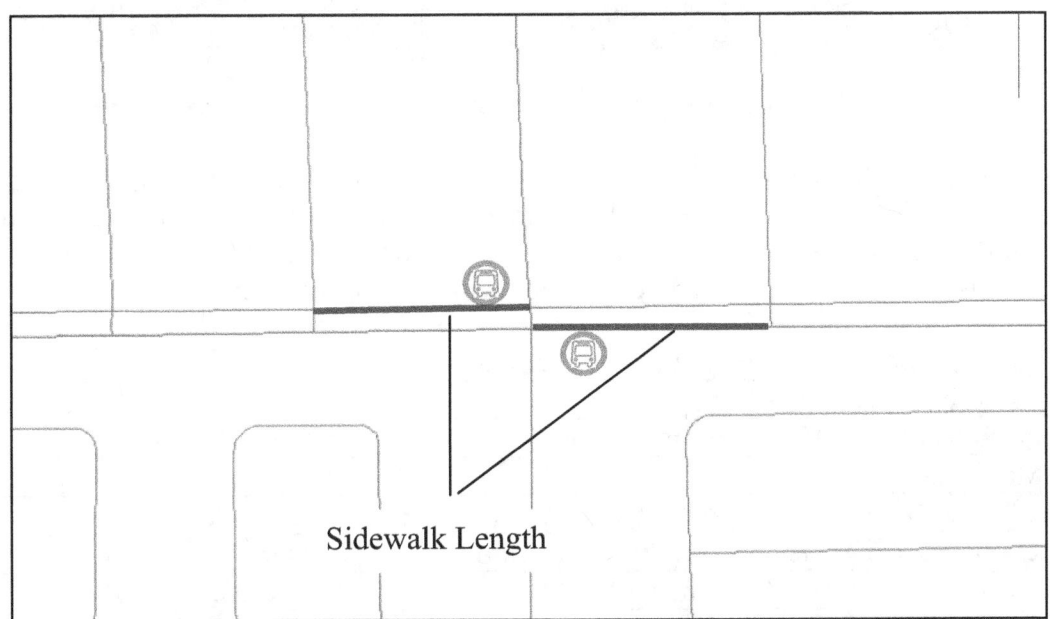

Figure 4-30 Calculation of Sidewalk Length.

As mentioned in Subsection 2.1.2, universal design will provide better quality services for people with disabilities. For the purposes of this research, improvements for universal design include shelters, benches, bus maps, and schedules. Shelter costs depend on building materials and additional facilities, such as transparent or opaque walls, heating, lighting and drainage. Shelters can cost up to $250,000 for major downtown locations. This research based its calculations on a common design with walls and general lighting equipment as shown in Figure 4-31; typically the cost for this design is around $5,000. Bench costs also vary if the design includes a back or armrests, with benches generally costing about $300. Furthermore, shelter sidewalk and pad construction must be estimated. The fields "SHELTER_PAD" and "All_Shelter_Sidewalk" provided information regarding whether the bus stop includes a sidewalk and/or a shelter pad, or does not. The general cost for a shelter sidewalk is about $300, and the cost for a shelter pad is around $500.

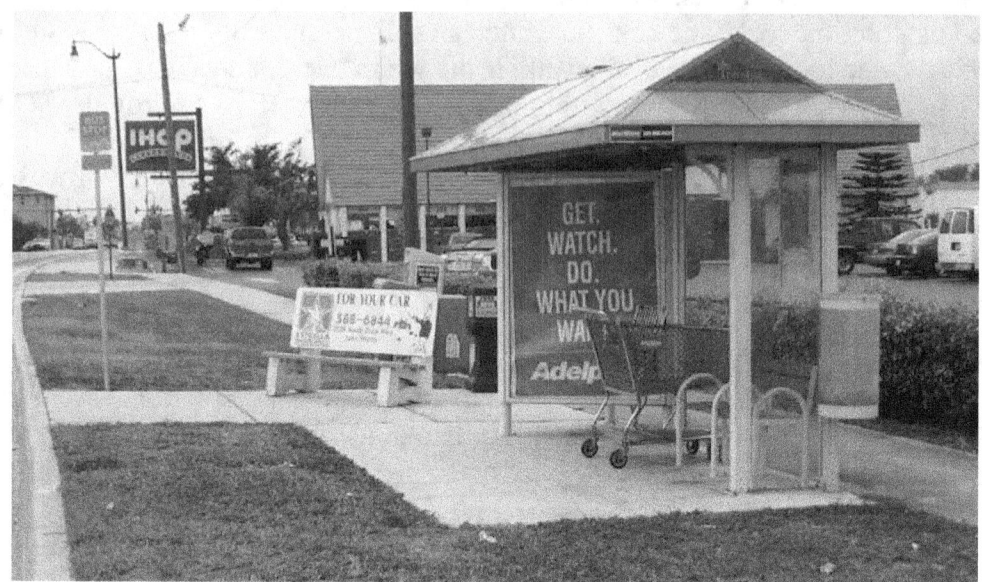

Figure 4-31 A Well-Designed Bus Stop Shelter in Broward County.

Table 4-9 illustrates the unit costs for various items with regard to ADA improvements at bus stops. Based on this cost information and the existing stop inventory, the total cost required to meet the minimum ADA and the universal design standards for each bus stop was calculated and available for use in the optimization model, which will be described next.

Table 4-9 Costs of ADA Bus Stop Improvements.

ADA Bus Stop Improvement Type	Unit	Unit Price
Survey, Mobilization and Labor Organization	Each	$500
Traffic Maintenance	Each	$500
Concrete Sidewalk, 6" Thick, 10-100 square yards	Square Yards	$54
Concrete Sidewalk, 6" Thick, 101-1000 square yards	Square Yards	$45
Concrete Curb, Type "D," 10-100 linear feet	Linear Feet	$11
Concrete Curb, Type "D," 101-1000 square yards	Linear Feet	$10
Subgrade Preparation for Concrete Pour	Square Yards	$2
Curb Cuts, Drawing I	Each	$800
Sidewalk Removal	Square Yards	$18
Curb Removal	Foot	$11
Improved Shelter with Roof, Walls and inside Lighting	Each	$5,000
Standard Bench	Each	$300
Bus Maps and Schedules	Each	$100

Table 4-10 summarizes the costs of bus stop improvements required to meet minimum ADA standards. It includes the number of bus stops and the average cost for each specific improvement. Sidewalk improvements require the largest investment. The average cost is about

$16,000 because the distance between the two nearest intersections can be quite long. Loading pads require the least construction work, so the average cost is only about $200. For all 2,465 candidate bus stops, the average cost for full improvements to meet minimum ADA standard is about $15,000.

Table 4-10 Summary: Cost of Bus Stop Improvements to Meet Minimum ADA Standards.

Improvement Type	The Number of Bus Stops	Average Cost per Bus Stop
For sidewalk improvement	1,663	$16,612.89
For curb cut improvement	1,969	$1,600.00
For loading pad improvement	2,267	$183.85
For all improvements	2,465	$15,360.82

Table 4-11 shows the summary of the improvement costs needed to meet universal design standards. The cost of the shelter is the sum of the price of the shelter itself and the relative construction fee. The average cost is around $6,300 for each candidate bus stop. Bench costs are fixed for each candidate bus stop, which is $300. For all 4,579 candidate bus stops, the average cost to make full improvements to meet universal design standards is around $6,500, which would be in addition to the $15,000 needed to meet minimum ADA standards.

Table 4-11 Summary: Cost of Bus Stop Improvements to Meet Universal Design Standards.

Improvement Type	The Number of Bus Stops	Average Cost per Bus Stop
For bench improvement	2,652	$300.00
For shelter improvement	4,565	$6,335.93
For all improvement	4,579	$6,500.25

4.9.3. Bus Stop Groups

Certain special situations arise that merit discussion with regard to costs. First, several candidate bus stops (usually two) share the same sidewalk that needs improvement, like the two red bus stops shown on Figure 4-32. Where bus stops share the same sidewalk, curb cuts are located at the nearest intersection, making it unnecessary to create additional curb cuts in the middle of the sidewalk. When the construction of several bus stops is performed at the same time, non-construction fees such as survey or labor organization could not be charged more than once. In other words, cost calculations would be duplicated if ADA improvement costs were built based on individual bus stop calculations because many stops share sidewalks, curb cut, and other costs. Economies of scale must be considered in the final analysis.

To avoid duplicate sidewalk improvement calculations, a dataset was developed for candidate bus stop groups using the following steps:

1. Calculate the sidewalk distance for each bus stop.
2. Group the bus stops that have the same sidewalk distance (suppose the sidewalk distance is unique for each sidewalk).
3. Filter the bus stop groups that have the same sidewalk distance based on the direction of the bus stop (ensure that the bus stops sharing the same sidewalk are on the same side of the road).

4. Use ArcGIS to inspect the bus stop and street network layer.

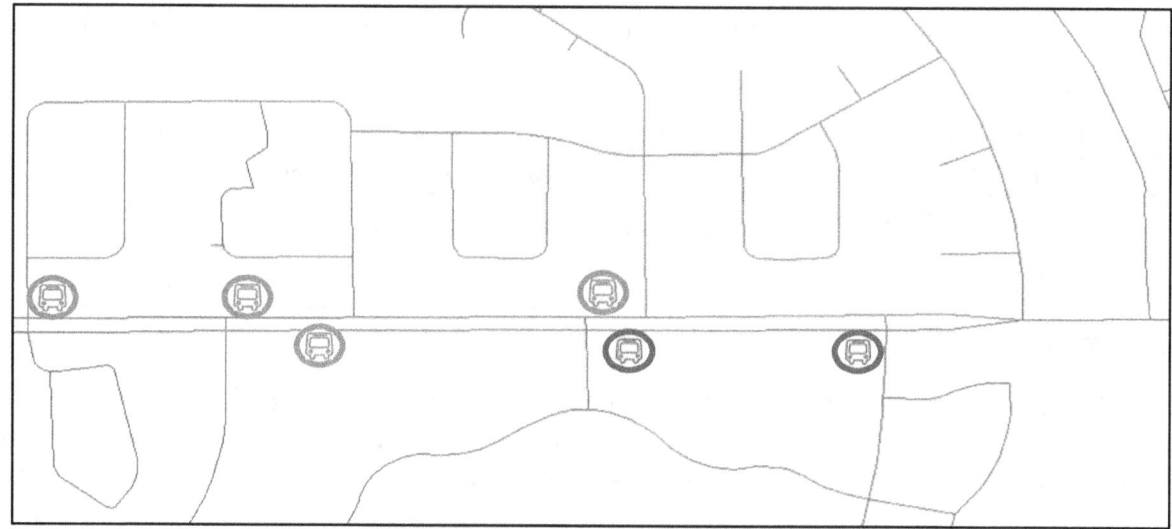

Figure 4-32 Bus Stops Sharing the Same Sidewalk.

The final list of candidate bus stop groups included 84 stop groups and 182 bus stops, in which 75 have two bus stops, six have three bus stops, two have four bus stops, and one has six bus stops. For each bus stop group, the cost of sidewalks, curb cuts, and the other non-construction fees were treated as the one single group cost, while the cost for loading pads was considered per bus stop and stored on the original bus top cost list.

4.10. Summary

In this chapter, the bus stop status inventory from Broward County Transit (BCT) was introduced as the base dataset for the data integration process. This inventory provides detailed accessibility information, which is especially important. Ridership data, including wheelchair boardings, general ridership based on bus stop location, and work trips by persons with disabilities, were taken into account. Socioeconomic factors, including population statistics regarding persons with disabilities as well as likely destinations and facilities were considered. The bus stop service area component was developed to integrate all the criteria. Factors that are interpreted as points were treated using a special arithmetic to solve the issue regarding closest distance in overlapping service areas. Finally, correlation analysis was performed to filter the factors that were highly correlated.

AHP was used to compare and evaluate eight different criteria within every candidate bus stop service area. The weights of different criteria were assigned by comparing and analyzing the travel patterns and percentage of riders with disabilities from Chapter 2. The weights may be different between minimum ADA standards and universal design standards because it is also the intention of universal design to benefit other bus riders. The ridership per stop that has been considered for universal design was assigned a higher weight than the corresponding minimum ADA standard level. Finally, the overall score of each candidate bus stop was standardized to evaluate the benefit to riders with disabilities. A user-friendly VBA program was developed to perform the calculations involved in all three stages, to make it easy for decision makers or planners to choose different weights based on their judgment and experience.

This chapter also presents the ADA improvement budget of Broward County and the construction cost estimates for candidate bus stops based on estimates from current contractors. Based on figures from the Broward County Transit Development Plan and the Broward County Metropolitan Planning Organization Transportation Improvement Program (Broward County Transit, 2005), the assigned budget—the main constraint of the optimization model—is $2.0 million per year between 2006 and 2010.

A full cost estimation list for each candidate bus stop was established. On this list, each bus stop has two different cost estimations based on both the minimum ADA standard and for the universal design standard. Besides the general cost for the survey, labor organization, and maintenance of traffic, the cost of bus stop improvements for the minimum ADA standard includes the sidewalk, loading pad, and curb cuts. The cost of bus stop improvements for universal design includes the bench, lighting, shelter, bus maps, and schedules. The final list of the candidate bus stops included 84 groups. This list was developed to avoid sidewalk length and curb cut calculation duplications, because 182 bus stops share the same sidewalk.

CHAPTER 5

OPTIMIZATION MODELS

Based on the literature review and the prescribed methodology, two standards have been established for bus stop improvements for riders with disabilities: the minimum ADA standards and the universal design standards. The minimum ADA standards provide the basic requirements needed to improve bus stops, while universal design requires a higher standard of improvement. In this chapter, two separate optimization models are developed. The first model aims to satisfy the minimum ADA standards while the second considers both the minimum ADA standards and the higher universal design standards.

5.1. Optimization Model for Minimum ADA Standards

The main objective for this optimization model is to maximize the overall benefits at the bus stop level (i.e., total R_i) to the riders with disabilities by making the minimum ADA improvements under the constraints of the available budget assigned to such improvements annually. The analytical hierarchy process (AHP) pre-processes all of the different criteria and generated one single weight for each candidate bus stop. This weight (R_i) then becomes the only standard by which to evaluate a given bus stop's importance with regard to accessibility improvements compared to the others. This method simplifies the final optimization model such that the objective function is the summation of R_i values of selected bus stops.

Within the constraints of this model, only complete ADA accessibility improvements were allowed for each bus stop. Single improvements, such as only building a loading pad without making other improvements, were not allowed in the optimization model. In other words, the transit agency could either choose to make full improvements or do nothing to a candidate bus stop. Another constraint stems from the limits of the available budget for ADA improvements.

A binary linear programming model was developed via a General Algebraic Modeling System (GAMS), version 2.50 (GAMS Development Corporation, 2007). GAMS is specifically designed for modeling linear, nonlinear, and mixed integer optimization problems. The system is especially useful with large, complex problems and provides users with great flexibility in programming. The optimization model being developed is relatively straightforward, but it has a large number of variables. GAMS is especially suited for solving these problems. Accordingly, the optimization model is defined below:

$$\max \sum_{i=1}^{n} R_i' y_i \tag{5-1}$$

subject to:

$$y_i \in \{0, 1\}$$
$$z_j \in \{0, 1\}$$

$$\sum_{i=1}^{n} c_i y_i + \sum_{j=1}^{m} c_j^s z_j < B$$

within dataset $d_g(i,j)$

$$z_j \leq \sum_{k=0}^{g-1} y_{i-k}$$

$$z_j \geq y_{i-k} \quad \forall\, k \in \{0, 1, \dots, g\text{-}1\}$$

where

R_i'	=	the standardized overall score of candidate bus stop i,
y_i	=	1 if candidate bus stop i is selected for improvements and 0 otherwise,
n	=	the total number of candidate bus stops,
c_i	=	the ADA improvement cost for candidate bus stop i (not including construction cost for sidewalk of bus stop groups),
z_j	=	1 if candidate bus stop group j is selected and 0 otherwise,
m	=	the total number of candidate bus stop groups,
c_j^s	=	the sidewalk improvement cost for candidate bus stop group j,
g	=	the number of bus stops within bus stop group (2, 3, 4 and 6),
$d_g(i,j)$	=	the corresponding relationship dataset between candidate bus stop i and bus stop group j, and
B	=	the total available budget for ADA improvements.

As explained in Subsection 4.9.3, a bus stop group consists of several candidate bus stops (usually two) that share the same sidewalk. The calculation of cost for a shared sidewalk will be duplicated if the ADA improvement cost is attributed to a single bus stop. Therefore, the cost estimation for each candidate bus stop is divided into two separate parts: c_i for the ADA improvement cost for candidate bus stop i (not including construction cost for sidewalk of bus stop groups); and c_j^s for the sidewalk improvement cost for candidate bus stop group j. To simplify the calculation, a total of 182 bus stops aggregated into groups were put at the top of the candidate bus stop list by the order of the length of shared sidewalk distance and the number of bus stops in bus stop group (from 2 to 6). Bus stops 1 to 150 were grouped into 75 bus stop groups with two bus stops; bus stops 151 to 168 were grouped into six bus stop groups with three bus stops; bus stops 169 to 176 were grouped into bus stop groups with four bus stops; bus stops 177 to 182 included six bus stops grouped together. For example, bus stops 1 and 2 were grouped together, and bus stops 151, 152 and 153 were grouped together.

The corresponding relationship dataset $d_g(i,j)$ was developed to build the relationship between candidate bus stop i and bus stop group j, in which g represents the number of bus stops within a bus stop group (2, 3, 4, 5, and 6). For example, $d_2(2,1)$ represents bus stop group 1 (including two bus stops) corresponding to bus stop 2, which is the last bus stop in bus stop group 1. Similarly, $d_3(153,76)$ represents bus stop group 76 (including three bus stops) corresponding to bus stop 153 which is the last bus stop in bus stop group 76.

In Equation 5-1, a binary variable z_j was introduced to prevent duplication of the improvement calculation. Taking bus stop group 1 as an example, three constraints were developed, i.e., $z_1 \leq$

$y_1 + y_2$, $z_1 \geq y_1$, and $z_1 \geq y_2$. If both y_1 and y_2 are zero, then $z_1 = 0$. If at least one of y_i is one, then $z_1 = 1$. Similarly, for bus stop group 76, four constraints were developed: $z_{76} \leq y_{151} + y_{152} + y_{153}$, $z_{76} \geq y_{151}$, $z_{76} \geq y_{152}$, and $z_{76} \geq y_{153}$. If y_{151}, y_{152} and y_{153} are all zero, then $z_{76} = 0$. If at least one of y_i is one, then $z_{76} = 1$. The duplicated improvement cost for each candidate bus stop group was based on the total ADA improvement cost if the candidate bus stop belongs to a bus stop group.

Given BCT's total available budget of \$2M for the next budget year and the associated construction costs, the output from the model shows that a total of 608 bus stops will get priority for ADA improvements for the next budget year. The maximum total R_i' is 3,321.13, and the total cost is \$1,999,476.

Because the bus stops with sidewalk improvements need much more investment than other candidate bus stops, the ratio of benefit over cost will be lower. Only 63 of the total 608 selected bus stops needed sidewalk improvements. The same applies to bus stop groups that share the same sidewalk; because those groups had a longer sidewalk, the cost for sidewalk improvement was more expensive than that for a single bus stop even if they share the cost of sidewalk improvements. Only two bus stop groups with the shortest shared sidewalk distance were kept in the final selected bus stop list. For this reason, a large number of bus stops (608 bus stops compared to the usual 300-500 bus stops every year) were selected. These calculations show that many bus stops need only minor investments to provide significant benefit to riders with disabilities. The maximum total R_i' and the number of selected bus stops are not the same for each budget year. The model will select bus stops with higher benefit-cost ratios for the current budget year and leaves the bus stops with lower benefit-cost ratios for the next year, so the maximum total R_i' and the number of selected bus stops will decline with each budget year, instead of the even improvement rate in the Broward County transit development plan.

Figure 5-1 shows the bus stops selected for ADA improvements as dark nodes. Compared to the distribution map of the population with disabilities, it clearly shows that the selected bus stops are generally located in those areas with a higher population with disabilities density—a criterion given the highest weight ($w_j = 0.3$) within the AHP process. The population with disabilities averages about 258 people living near the selected bus stops compared to an average population with disabilities of about 175 for the remaining bus stops. The significance of bus ridership ($w_j = 0.2$) is also reflected in the final map in Figure 5-1 when compared to the ridership map in Figure 4-23. The average ridership is 917.37 for the selected bus stops versus 676.25 for the rest. Those bus stop locations match the distribution of health care facilities, religious centers, parks, schools, and shopping centers. Note that, for practical purposes, it is convenient to group these bus stops and make ADA improvements to all of them because they are so close together.

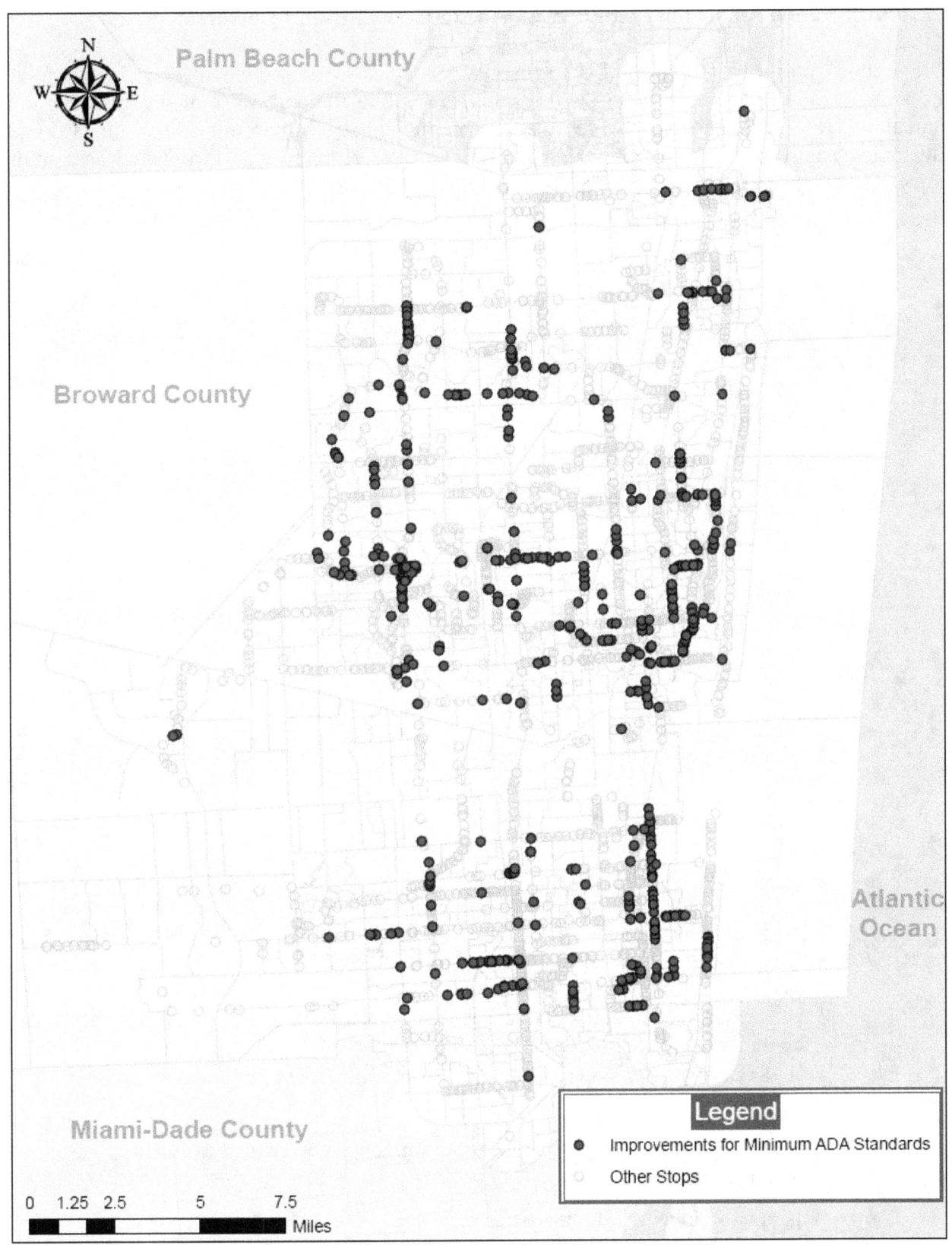

Figure 5-1 Selected Bus Stops for ADA Improvements.

5.2. Optimization Model for Minimum ADA Improvements and Universal Design

The second optimization model seeks to identify bus stops for improvements that will result in the largest overall benefits to riders with disabilities within the constraint of the available total annual budget. Two objectives were considered: meeting the minimum ADA standards and meeting the universal design standards. Accordingly, the problem was formulated as a multi-objective binary nonlinear program, defined as follows:

$$Max \sum_{i=1}^{n} R_i' y_i \tag{5-2}$$

$$Max \sum_{i=1}^{n} (P_i' x_i y_i + Q_i' x_i) \tag{5-3}$$

subject to

$$x_i \in \{0,1\}$$

$$y_i \in \{0,1\}$$

$$z_j \in \{0,1\}$$

$$\sum_{i=0}^{n} (c_i y_i + b_i x_i) + \sum_{j=1}^{m} c_j^s z_j \leq B$$

within dataset $d_g(i,j)$

$$z_j \leq \sum_{k=0}^{g-1} y_{i-k}$$

$$z_j \geq y_{i-k} \quad \forall\, k \in \{0, 1, \ldots, g\text{-}1\}$$

where

R_i' = the standardized overall score based on minimum ADA standards for bus stop i,

P_i' = the standardized overall score based on universal design for bus stop i that do not meet the minimum ADA standards,

Q_i' = the standardized overall score based on universal design for bus stop i that meets the minimum ADA standards,

y_i = $\begin{cases} 1 \text{ if candidate bus stop } i \text{ is selected for minimum ADA improvement,} \\ 0 \text{ otherwise,} \end{cases}$

x_i = $\begin{cases} 1 \text{ if candidate bus stop } i \text{ is selected for universal design improvement,} \\ 0 \text{ otherwise,} \end{cases}$

n = the total number of candidate bus stops,

b_i = the required ADA improvement cost based on universal design for candidate bus stop i,

m = the total number of candidate bus stop groups,

c_i = the required ADA improvement cost based on minimum ADA standards for candidate bus stop i,

c_j^s = the sidewalk improvement cost for candidate bus stop group,

$d_g(i, j)$ = the corresponding relationship dataset between candidate bus stop i and bus stop group j, and

B = the total available budget for ADA improvements.

Similar to the single-goal optimization model for meeting the minimum ADA standards, the data set $d_g(i, j)$, binary variable z_j, and several constraints were introduced to prevent duplicate cost calculations.

Again, the AHP pre-processed all of the different criteria and generated a single score for each bus stop. The three total scores, R_i', P_i' and Q_i', then became the standards by which to determine the importance of ADA improvements at a given bus stop relative to other bus stops. This simplifies the final optimization model by allowing the objective function value to be the summation of the R_i', P_i' and Q_i', values of the selected bus stops. Using the goal programming approach, the equation below was transformed into a single objective model by introducing two goal deviations, d_1 and d_2, defined as:

$$Min \ (d_1 + d_2) \tag{5-4}$$

subject to

$$x_i \in \{0,1\}$$

$$y_i \in \{0,1\}$$

$$z_j \in \{0,1\}$$

$$d_1, d_2 \geq 0$$

$$\sum_{i=1}^{n} R_i' y_i + d_1 \geq t_d$$

$$\sum_{i=1}^{n} (P_i' x_i y_i + Q_i' x_i) + d_2 \geq t_u$$

$$\sum_{i=1}^{n} (c_i y_i + b_i x_i) + \sum_{j=1}^{m} c_j^s z_j \leq B$$

within dataset $d^g(i, j)$

$$z_j \leq \sum_{k=0}^{g-1} y_{i-k}$$

$$z_j \geq y_{i-k} \quad \forall \, k \in \{0, 1, \ldots, g\text{-}1\}$$

where

d_1 = goal deviation for minimum ADA improvements,

d_2 = goal deviation for universal design improvements,

t_d = target level for minimum ADA improvements, and

t_u = target level for universal design improvements.

(The other variables are as defined previously.)

In the goal programming alternative, d_1 and d_2 are positive goal deviations to achieve an optimal compromise between the two different objectives. An optimal compromise among the different objectives is then derived to minimize the deviations from the goals, t_d and t_u, the target levels for the two objectives to be achieved. They also reflect the fact that the importance of any objective diminishes once a target level has been achieved.

This formulation assumes that the selected bus stops will fully meet ADA accessibility requirements. Single improvements, such as building only a loading pad or a bench while other improvements are not made, were not allowed in each objective. The constraints were discrete binary constraints—they either made all the improvements or they did not. For the two-objective optimization, the transit agency could either choose to fully meet the requirements or do nothing to a candidate bus stop. For the universal design level optimization, building a shelter at the bus stop that does not meet the minimum ADA standard is not meaningful, so the candidate bus stops for the universal design were selected from the bus stops that have already been selected based on the minimum ADA standards. Another constraint stems from the limits of the total available budget for ADA improvements.

In Equations (5-2) and (5-3), R_i' and P_i' will be 0 for those bus stops that already meet the minimum ADA standards, and Q_i' will be 0 for those bus stops that already meet minimum ADA standards but not the universal design standards. This prevents the model from selecting bus stops that have a high score but do not need any ADA improvements. The term z_iy_i was included to ensure that the bus stops selected for universal design improvements were selected from those that have met the minimum ADA requirements.

The multi-objective model was developed based on CoinBonmin 0.9 (Basic Open-source Nonlinear Mixed Integer programming) via the General Algebraic Modeling System (GAMS), version 2.50.

Given BCT's total available budget of \$2M for the next budget year and the associated construction costs, the initial t_d and t_u should be assigned to the model (decision-makers can change the two values easily and adjust the importance comparing the two objectives). Because the model is a nonlinear mixed integer programming, it cannot ensure that every combination of t_d and t_u has a feasible solution. Based on the maximum total R_i' from optimization model for minimum ADA improvements, the model calculated different combinations of t_d and t_u for a sum of around 3200. Table 5-1 shows the model output of different combination of t_d and t_u. Notice that under the combination of $t_d = 3200$ and $t_u = 0$, 13 bus stops were still assigned to meet universal design improvement standards, and that no feasible solution covers all areas in combination. The single objective model was still the best choice if it is only possible to choose the minimum ADA standard improvements.

Table 5-1 Model Output with Different Combinations of t_d and t_u.

t_d	t_u	d_1	d_2	Number of bus stops for Min ADA Standard	Number of bus stops for Universal Design
3200	0	0	0	561	13
3300	0	0	0	599	13
3400	0	-	-	-	-
3100	200	0	0	539	45
3200	200	-	-	-	-
3000	300	0	5.69	529	61
3100	300	-	-	-	-
2900	**500**	**4.82**	**52.98**	**510**	**77**
2500	700	0	1.15	424	132
2700	700	-	-	-	-
2200	900	0	10.51	373	173
2300	900	5.15	59.08	392	161
2400	900	-	-	-	-
1200	1200	-	-	-	-
1500	1200	6.57	60.79	226	237
1000	1400	-	-	-	-

The initial defaults for t_d and t_a were equal to 2900 and 500 in this model. The output from the model shows that a total of 549 bus stops get priority with regard to ADA improvements for the next budget year, in which 510 bus stops need minimum ADA improvements, 77 bus stops need universal design improvements, and 38 bus stops need both minimum ADA improvements and universal design improvements. The minimum total d_1+d_2 is 57.8, and the total cost is $1,999,975. Figure 5-2 shows the bus stops selected for ADA improvement as dark nodes.

Table 5-2 Average Ridership Comparison for Selected Bus Stops.

Average Ridership	Selected for Minimum ADA Improvements	Selected for Universal Design Improvements
825.27	No	No
3758.66	No	Yes
895.04	Yes	No
1390.14	Yes	Yes

The selected bus stops are generally located in those areas with a higher ridership in comparison to the ridership distribution map because the ridership criterion gets the highest weight (w_j=0.35) within the AHP system. The average ridership comparison for selected bus stops and the rest are shown in Table 5-2. Because those bus stops that have already met the minimum ADA standards usually have a higher ridership, the bus stops that were selected for universal design improvements also have a higher ridership, as is indicated in Table 5-2. The bus stops that were selected for both minimum ADA standards and universal design improvements represent a compromise, such that the average ridership is relatively lower when compared to those selected for universal design improvements only. Naturally, the bus stops that were not selected for either improvement have the lowest average ridership. Comparing Figure 4-29 with Figure 5-2 illustrates that the selected bus stops also match the distribution trends of the standardized overall score R'. Note that, for practical purposes, it is convenient to group these bus stops and make ADA improvements to all of them because they are so close together.

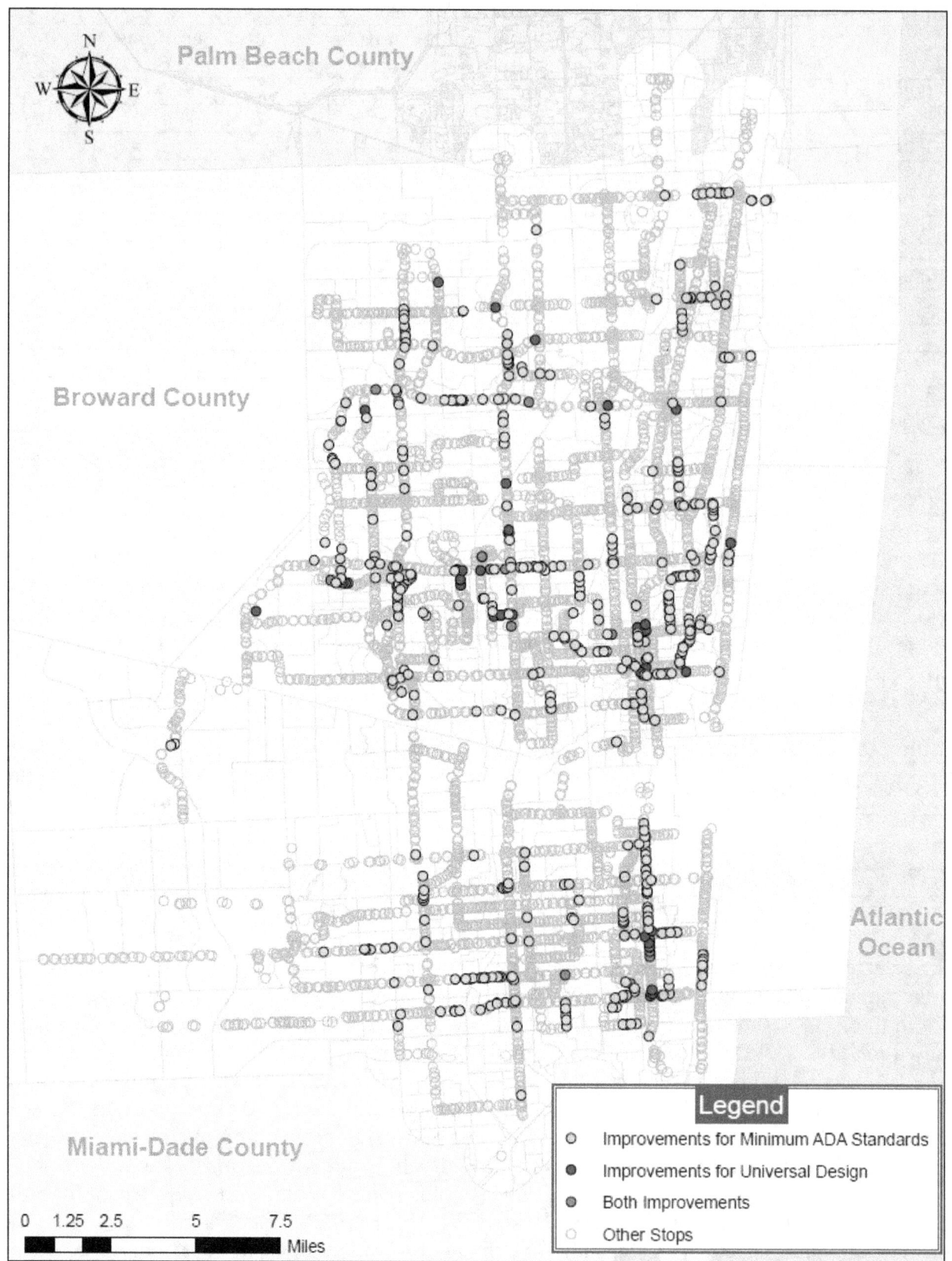

Figure 5-2 Selected Bus Stops for ADA Improvements and Universal Design.

5.3. Summary

In this chapter, two different optimization models were developed for ADA bus stop improvements to meet different objectives: 1) satisfying the minimum ADA standard, and 2) satisfying both objectives—the minimum ADA standard and the higher universal design standard. The former is a comparatively simple binary linear programming model, and the latter mainly applies a nonlinear mixed integer model in goal programming via the General Algebraic Modeling System (GAMS). GAMS is specifically suited to these two optimization models.

In the two optimization models, the corresponding relationship dataset between a candidate bus stop and a bus stop group was introduced to prevent duplication in cost calculation for sidewalk and curb-cut construction. The models assume that the selected bus stops will be made to fully meet the ADA accessibility requirements or the universal design requirements. Single improvements, such as building only a loading pad or a bench, are not allowed in each objective.

From the model output based on the BCT data, about 600 bus stops were selected for ADA improvement for the next funding cycle. The results show that a large percentage of the selected bus stops needed only minor investments to substantially benefit riders with disabilities. Because the model is a nonlinear mixed integer programming, it cannot ensure that every combination has a feasible solution. The single objective model is preferred if only the minimum ADA standards need to be met.

These two optimization models have different applicability. Based on the Broward County bus stop accessibility inventory, nearly half of the bus stops did not meet minimum ADA requirements; some of them only need a minor investment to meet the minimum ADA requirements. Meeting the minimum ADA requirements should be the priority (rather than making the investment to meet the universal design standard) due to the limited County budget. Therefore, the single objective model that aims to meet the minimum ADA standard was more suitable for Broward County. On the other hand, if a large number of the bus stops for a transit agency were qualified under the minimum ADA standard, that agency might be able to improve the accessibility of bus stops at the higher service level standard. The second model that aims to satisfy two objectives would thusly be a better choice.

CHAPTER 6

SENSITIVITY ANALYSIS

After model optimization, sensitivity analysis is used to identify how input changes (the ratio among the factors and the change in the budget) affect model outputs. It helps decision makers learn how the various decision elements interact to determine the most preferred alternative, as well as which elements are important sources of disagreement among the decision makers. Because it is difficult to perform sensitivity analysis on a nonlinear programming model, all these sensitivity analyses are based on the optimization model only for the minimum ADA improvements.

6.1. Budget Sensitivity Analysis

Figure 6-1 shows the change in total R' and the number of selected bus stops if the budget is changed from $10,000 to $3,000,000. Both curves can be seen to change smoothly with no obvious break points. The decreasing rate of the curves suggests that the benefit-cost ratios are higher when the budget is low. As explained in Chapter 5.2, the model will select those bus stop with higher R' and lower improvement costs (for example, where no sidewalk improvement is needed). Accordingly, the total R' and the number of selected bus stops initially increase more rapidly. As the budget increases, more bus stops with higher R' but a more expensive investment rate will be selected, causing the curve to become flatter.

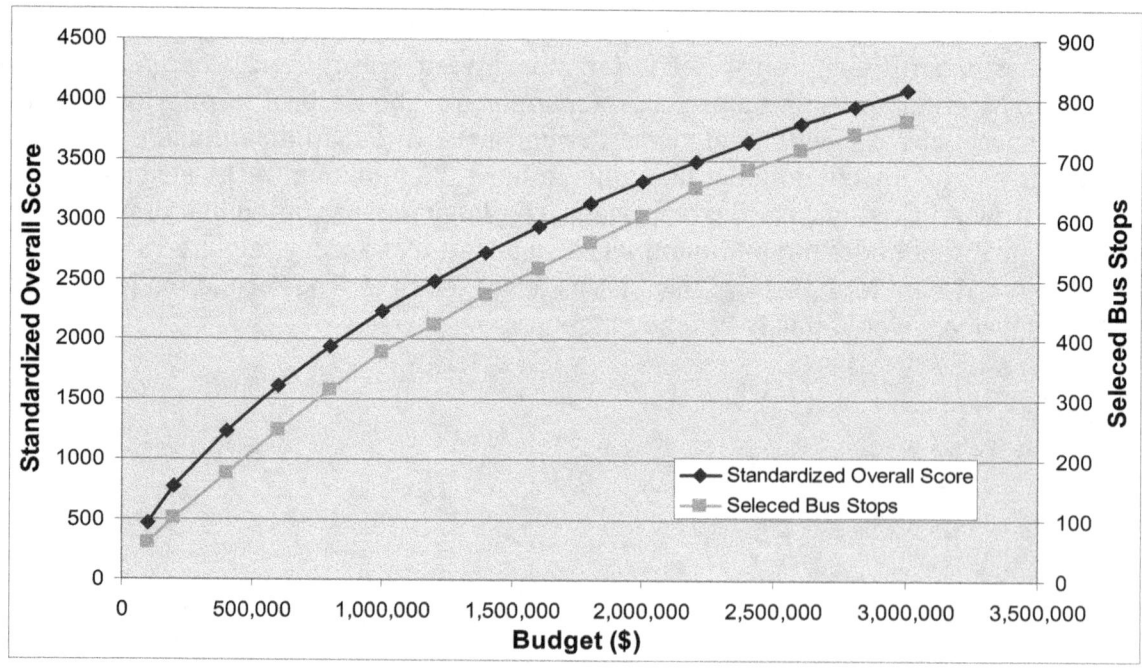

Figure 6-1 Budget Sensitivity Analysis.

6.2. Factor Sensitivity Analysis

This analysis examines the sensitivity of output to changes in the weight for each of the eight factors considered in this research. The weight w_j is a very significant coefficient because it reflects the importance among all the factors. In practice, the decision maker may change the default value of w_j based on his/her experience or the real situation. For this reason, we must know how the change of w_j for each factor affects the total model output.

Table 6-1 and Figure 6-2 illustrate how the change in the weight value w_j for religious centers affects the final output. The default value is 0.035; about 30 bus stops changed positions from the total selected bus stops when w_j increased by 0.1. Total R' also increased as the w_j increased, and the number of total selected bus stops decreased as w_j increased, because as w_j increases, only the bus stops near religious centers will be weighted higher. The location of religious centers limits the number of affected bus stops. If the total R' were kept at the same level, the number of total selected bus stops should decrease.

Table 6-1 Change in Weights for Religious Centers.

w_j	Number of Bus Stops				Total R'
	Total change	New selected	Not included	Total selected	
0.035	0	0	0	608	3321.13
0.1	30	14	16	606	3320.77
0.2	63	25	38	595	3341.69
0.3	92	36	56	588	3365.94
0.4	124	46	78	576	3404.46
0.5	150	56	94	570	3446.72

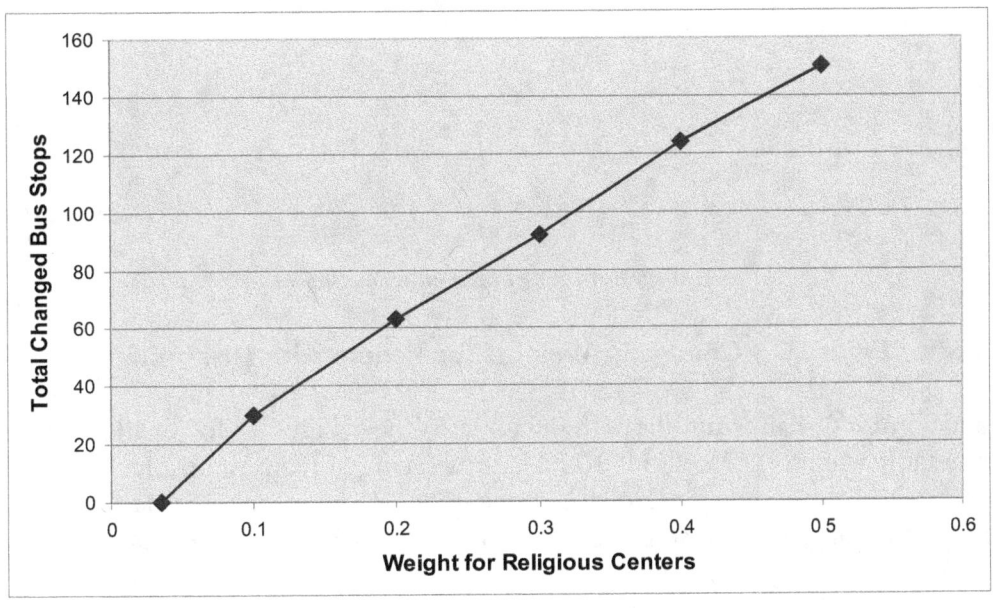

Figure 6-2 Change in Weights for Religious Centers.

Table 6-2 and Figure 6-3 show the change in the weight w_j for the distribution of the population with disabilities. The default value is 0.30; about 20 bus stops changed positions from the total number of selected bus stops when w_j increased by 0.1, and 35 bus stops changed when w_j changed from 0.3 to 0.2. Basically, the total R' and the total selected bus stops stayed the same while the weight w_j changed. Minor changes were caused by the relatively even distribution of persons with disabilities compared to the additional factors—the other reason is that the default value for w_j for this population's distribution was already high.

Table 6-2 Change in Weights for People with Disabilities.

w_j	Number of Bus Stops				Total R'
	Total change	New selected	Not included	Total selected	
0.2	35	18	17	609	3334.89
0.3	0	0	0	608	3321.13
0.4	30	14	16	606	3311.62
0.5	45	21	24	605	3310.23
0.6	54	26	28	606	3311.22
0.7	66	31	35	604	3312.83

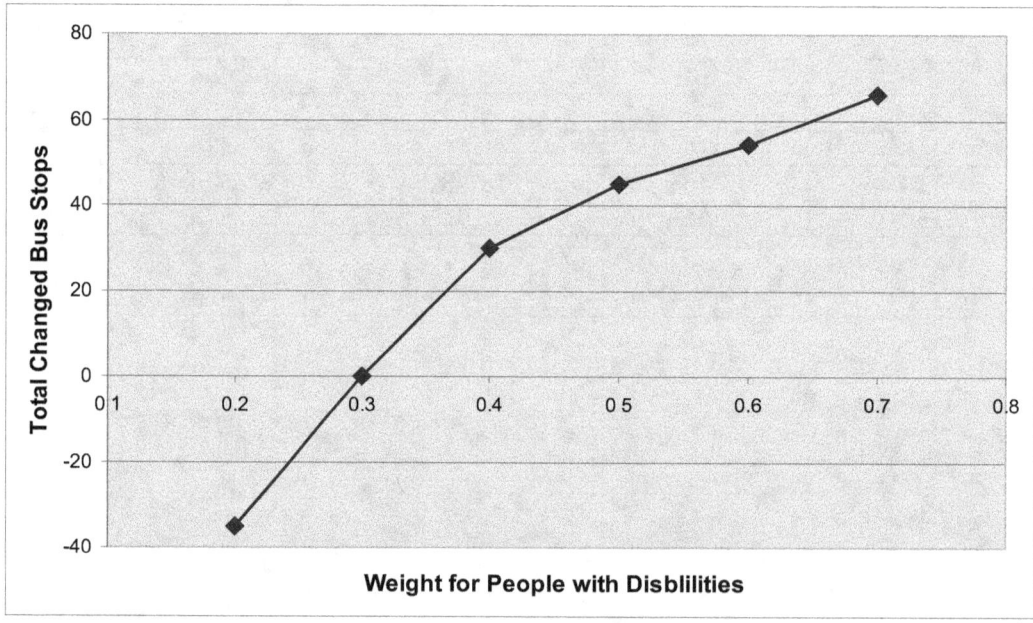

Figure 6-3 Change in Weights for People with Disabilities

Table 6-3 and Figure 6-4 illustrate how the change in the weight w_j for health centers alters the output. The default value is 0.05; about 30 bus stops changed from total selected bus stops when w_j increased by 0.1. Similar to religious centers, total R' increases a little when w_j increases; subsequently, the number of total selected bus stops decreases as w_j increases.

Table 6-3 Change in Weights for Health Centers.

w_j	Number of Bus Stops				Total R'
	Total change	New selected	Not included	Total selected	
0.05	33	15	18	605	3304.43
0.1	0	0	0	608	3321.13
0.2	44	24	20	612	3360.8
0.3	77	37	40	605	3424.71
0.4	103	46	57	597	3486.65
0.5	132	54	78	584	3550.14

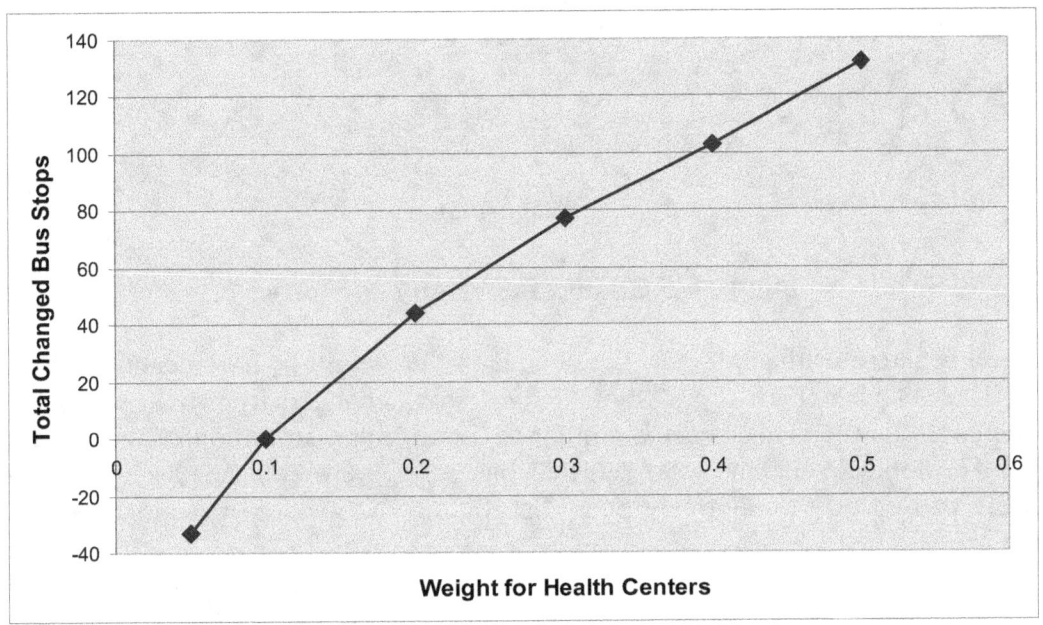

Figure 6-4 Change in Weights for Health Centers.

Table 6-4 and Figure 6-5 illustrate how the change of w_j for parks affects the final output. The default value is 0.035; about 16 bus stops changed from the total number of selected bus stops when w_j increased by 0.1. Basically, the total R' and the total number of selected bus stops were constant while w_j changed because Broward County has fewer parks and a higher incidence of other facilities; even as the weight w_j increases, the weights of most bus stops were decided by other factors which resulted in small changes to the output.

Table 6-4 Change in Weights for Parks.

w_j	Number of Bus Stops				Total R'
	Total change	New selected	Not included	Total selected	
0.035	0	0	0	608	3321.13
0.1	16	10	6	612	3307.16
0.2	29	15	14	609	3310.19
0.3	43	20	23	605	3290.95
0.4	73	29	44	593	3292.83
0.5	89	34	55	587	3300.58

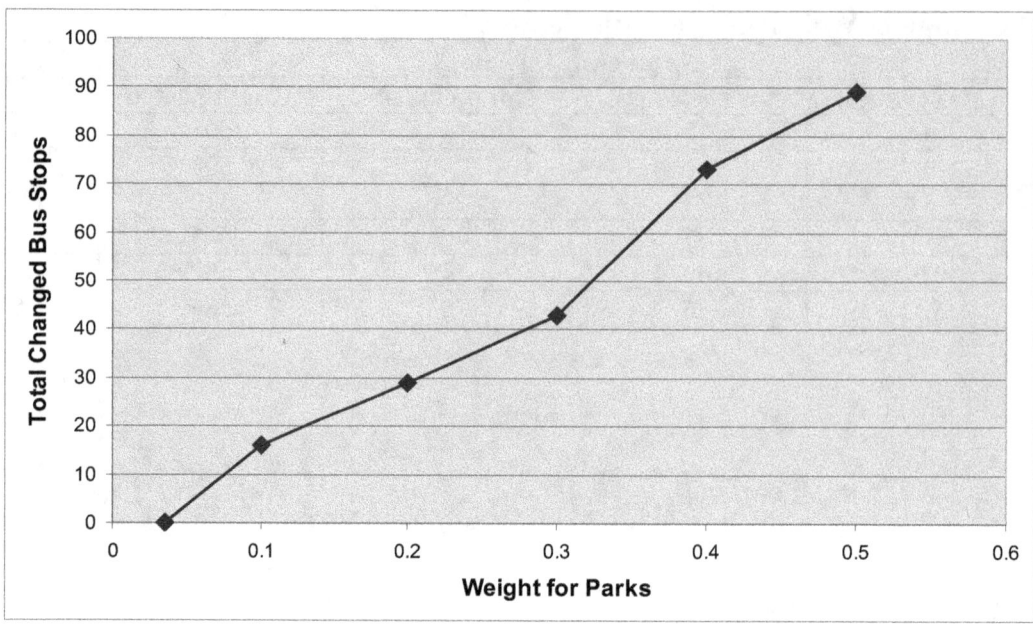

Figure 6-5 Change in Weights for Parks.

Table 6-5 and Figure 6-6 illustrate how the change in the weight w_j for ridership per stop affects the output. The default value is 0.20; about 10 bus stops changed from total selected bus stops when w_j increased by 0.1. This affect is similar to that of the distribution of the population with disabilities. The total R' and the total selected bus stops were constant as w_j changed. Minor changes were caused by the relatively even distribution of ridership per stop compared to the other factors.

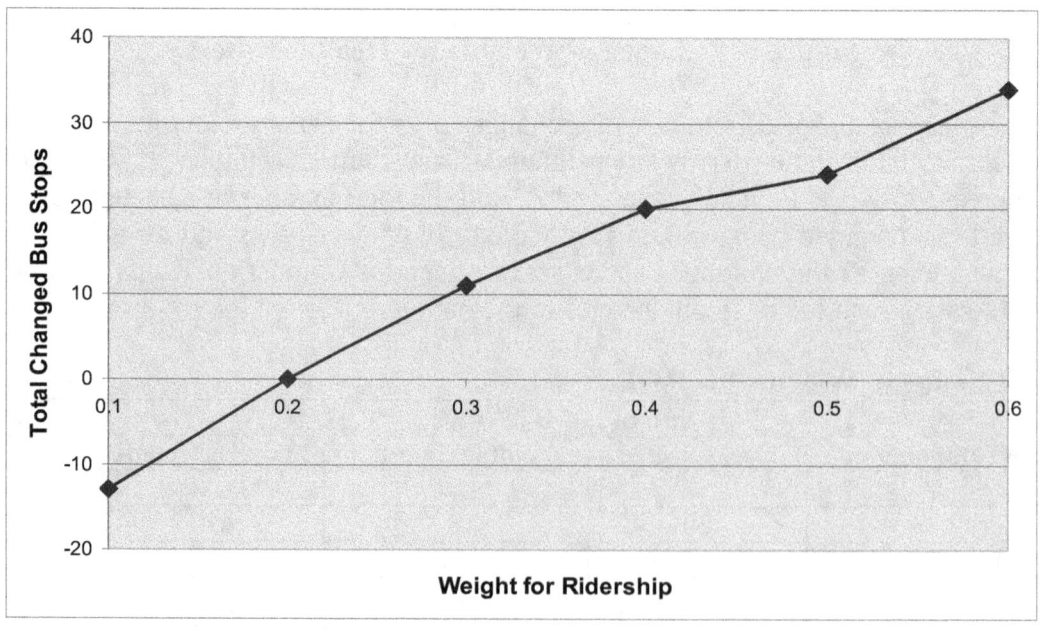

Figure 6-6 Change in Weights for Ridership.
Table 6-5 Change in Weights for Ridership.

w_j	Number of Bus Stops				Total R'
	Total change	New selected	Not included	Total selected	
0.1	13	6	7	609	3340.69
0.2	0	0	0	608	3321.13
0.3	11	7	4	606	3320.77
0.4	20	10	10	595	3341.69
0.5	24	12	12	588	3365.94
0.6	34	16	18	576	3404.46

Table 6-6 and Figure 6-7 illustrate how the change in the weight w_j for schools affects the total output. The default value is 0.10; about 30 bus stops changed from total selected bus stops when w_j increased by 0.1. Like religious centers, the total R' increases slightly as w_j increases, and the number of total selected bus stops decreases as w_j increases.

Table 6-6 Change in Weights for Schools.

w_j	Number of Bus Stops				Total R'
	Total change	New selected	Not included	Total selected	
0.05	32	18	14	612	3309.55
0.1	0	0	0	608	3321.13
0.2	41	17	24	601	3355.82
0.3	74	28	46	590	3404.32
0.4	96	36	60	584	3459.63
0.5	115	41	74	575	3516.25

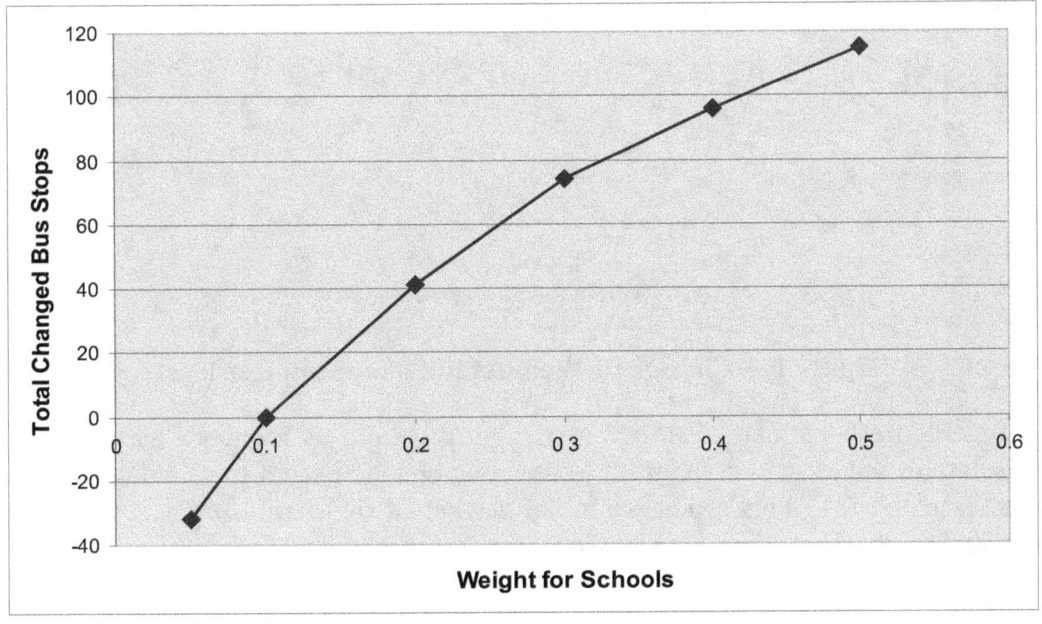

Figure 6-7 Change in Weights for Schools.

Table 6-7 and Figure 6-8 illustrate how the change in weight w_j for shopping centers affects the total output. The default value is 0.10; about 20 bus stops changed from the total selected bus stops when w_j increases by 0.1. The total R' and total selected bus stops are constant as w_j increases.

Table 6-7 Change in Weights for Shopping Centers.

w_j	Number of Bus Stops				Total R'
	Total change	New selected	Not included	Total selected	
0.08	0	0	0	608	3321.13
0.2	31	16	15	609	3329.51
0.3	44	22	22	608	3341.89
0.4	63	29	34	603	3357.18
0.5	83	35	48	595	3372.84
0.6	94	40	54	594	3393.95

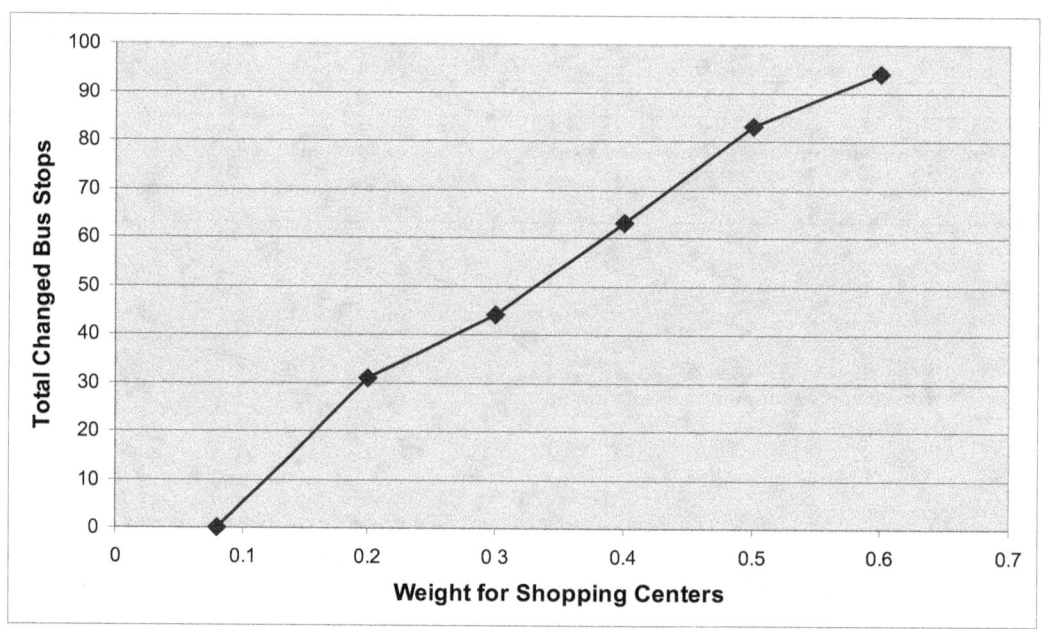

Figure 6-8 Change in Weights for Shopping Centers.

Table 6-8 and Figure 6-9 illustrate how the change in weight w_j for work trips affects the total output. The default value is 0.15; about 20 bus stops changed from the total selected bus stops when w_j increases by 0.1. This affect is similar to that of the distribution of shopping centers. The total R' and total selected bus stops are constant as w_j increases.

Table 6-8 Change in Weights for Work Trips.

| w_j | Number of Bus Stops | | | | Total R' |
	Total change	New selected	Not included	Total selected	
0.05	25	14	11	611	3332.36
0.15	0	0	0	608	3321.13
0.25	23	13	10	611	3312.28
0.35	40	22	18	612	3307.96
0.45	62	29	33	604	3309.38
0.55	75	34	41	601	3313.85

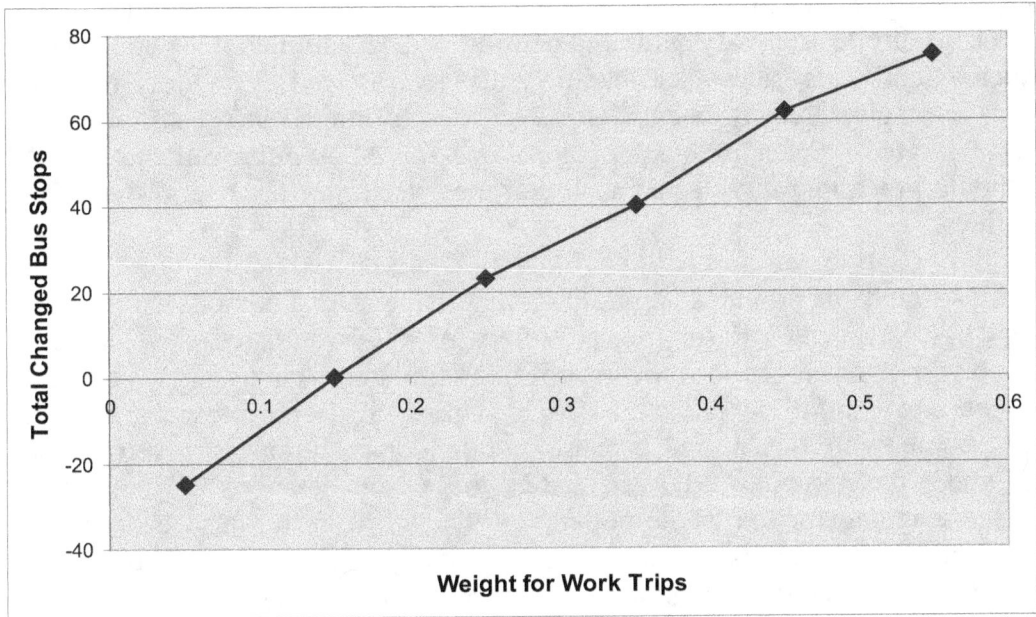

Figure 6-9 Change in Weights for Work Trips.

6.3. Summary

The sensitivity analysis performed in this chapter shows that the optimization models presented in Chapter 5 are reasonable. The budget sensitivity analysis describes how the model is more efficient when the budget is lower because the model selected as many bus stops as possible with higher scores at lower cost. When the budget is higher, the benefit-cost ratios of the remaining candidate bus stops should be lower, so the efficiency of the model will be lower. It also explains why over 600 bus stops were selected for improvement during next budget year. As BCT makes progress improving bus stops to meet ADA standards, the number of selected bus stops will decrease each year.

Factor sensitivity analysis was utilized to inspect how the changes in the weights for each factor will affect the optimization model. The model output shows that there were no break points for the factors—every weighted curve changed smoothly. When the ratio of each factor increased by 0.1, the model selected bus stops changed by 10 to 35 bus stops, while the total score basically remained constant. Compared to the other factors, religious centers, health centers, and schools caused larger changes to the optimization model.

CHAPTER 7

SUMMARY, CONCLUSIONS, AND RECOMMENDATIONS

7.1. Summary

Inaccessible bus stops prevent people with disabilities from using fixed-route bus services, thus limiting their mobility. The Americans with Disabilities Act (ADA) of 1990 prescribes the minimum requirements for bus stop accessibility by riders with disabilities. Although the accessibility improvements mandated under the ADA have enforceable regulations and standards, many bus stops still do not meet the mandate. Clearly, one way for transit agencies to improve accessibility to transit systems for patrons with disabilities is to add ADA-compliant features such as curb cuts, sidewalks, loading pads, etc., as well as auditory messages such as talking signs and voice announcements. However, due to limited budgets, transit agencies can only select a limited number of bus stop locations for ADA improvements annually. These locations should preferably be selected such that they maximize the overall benefits to patrons with disabilities.

While the ADA standards provide the minimum requirements that comply with law, they are not necessarily "best practices." Easter Seals Project ACTION initiated the "universal design" concept for bus stops. The goal of universal design is to create environments that facilitate bus access, safety, and comfort for all transit users. Universal design provides a higher level of access for people with disabilities because, while consideration is given to people with disabilities under the minimum ADA standards, these considerations are not sufficient when planning and designing for the whole population. Universal design also benefits other people with reduced mobility, such as children, older adults, parents pushing strollers, people with temporary injuries, pregnant women, and even travelers pulling luggage. Universal design is a better choice than ADA minimum requirements if the public transit planning or improvement project has the requisite budget.

The goal of this research was to develop a decision-making tool that can better identify the types of improvements needed and to determine the most effective locations for these improvements under budget constraints. The specific objectives of this research are:

1. Establish a bus stop requirement checklist based on minimum ADA and universal design standards for riders with disabilities.
2. Develop a database that includes bus stop inventory, transit ridership, transit budget, and socioeconomic data; determine the constraints; and standardize the various evaluation criteria.
3. Develop two optimization models to help identify a priority list of bus stops for accessibility improvements, one to meet only the minimum ADA requirements, and a second to achieve an optimal compromise among the minimum ADA and universal design standards.

A comprehensive literature review was conducted to investigate and assess the current standards for bus stop improvements for riders with disabilities in terms of meeting the minimum ADA and universal design standards. The literature search and review also involved the state-of-the-art techniques and research regarding transit accessibility. Public transit pattern studies for persons with disabilities were reviewed. Transit service optimization and relevant issues such as transit service accessibility models and uniform density problems in the GIS buffer analysis were reviewed. As the major method, spatial multicriteria decision making and its applications in transportation-related problems were fully reviewed.

Broward County Transit (BCT) provided a bus stop status inventory that includes data on 5,034 bus stops. Using this inventory, a full checklist was developed to evaluate current bus stop conditions for riders with disabilities based on the ADA minimum requirements and universal design standards. Data from different sources, including Broward County Transit, Florida Geographic Data Library and Census Transportation Planning Package, were collected. A total of eight factors (bus ridership data, disabilities census data, and various facilities' locational data) were organized to generate data for evaluation criteria. Bus stop service area based on the street network was selected as the basic unit of analysis. A unified database that integrated bus stop status with the other criteria was developed within the bus stop service area.

The analytical hierarchy process (AHP) was then used to combine and generate overall weights for every bus stop given the different factors and criteria. A user-friendly VBA program was developed to perform all the calculations involved in the above three stages, to make it easy for decision makers or planners to choose different vector of priority weights based on their judgment and experience.

After budget and cost estimation for various ADA bus stop improvements, two different optimization models were developed. One only considered satisfying the minimum ADA standard, while the other took the objectives for both the minimum ADA standards and universal design into account. A detailed sensitivity analysis was performed to evaluate bus stop selection based on changes in the budget as well as changes in the weights for the various factors. The analysis was used to identify how the ratio among the factors and the change of the budget affect the model outputs. This analysis tested the optimization model to determine if the model was robust or if the decision maker should review the evaluation criteria step to re-evaluate any needed changes. This procedure will help decision makers learn how the various decision elements interact to determine the most preferred alternative, as well as which elements are important sources of disagreement. The sensitivity analysis output in Chapter 6 showed the optimization model is reasonable and robust for the bus stop improvements studied here.

7.2. Conclusions

In this research, a GIS-based decision support system was developed for allocating bus stop facility improvements for riders with disabilities using Broward County Transit data. First, a full bus stop accessibility checklist for riders with disabilities accessibility was developed based on an analysis of the ADA minimum requirements and universal design standards. The construction cost was also estimated for every candidate bus stop.

The research and literature review on public transit pattern study for the population of people with disabilities revealed that the evaluation criteria covered almost every type of journey of riders with disabilities, from the distribution of the population with disabilities to potential destination places (health centers, shopping centers, schools, and so on). Ridership data based on each bus top was introduced to accurately evaluate its utilization rate; ridership data cannot be the only evaluation criteria because it does not fully reflect all the journeys that riders with disabilities make by bus. In addition, intentionally improving bus stop accessibility by utilizing the distribution of the population with disabilities and their most popular destinations may stimulate ridership in the community with disabilities. The distance decay model, short distance calculation, and service area were introduced to better specify the bus stop service area and service quality analysis.

By evaluating eight different criteria within every candidate bus stop service area, the analytical hierarchy process (AHP) calculated a single scenario with one simple number. This method has the advantage of simplifying the final optimization model and giving the decision maker a straightforward idea of which bus stops should have priority in building ADA improvements. The vector of weighted priorities could be established freely to meet the requirements based on the minimum ADA or universal design standards. A user-friendly VBA program was developed to perform all the calculations involved in all three stages, and to give decision makers and planners maximum flexibility to choose different vectors of priorities based on their judgment and experience.

In this research, two different optimization models were developed for ADA bus stop improvements to meet different objectives. One only considered satisfying the minimum ADA standards, while the other took into account two objectives—the minimum ADA standards and the higher standard of universal design. Based on the model output, about 600 bus stops need ADA improvements during the next budget year. Fewer bus stops needing sidewalk improvements were selected because of their higher investment. A large portion of selected bus stops require only minor investments to greatly benefit riders with disabilities. The multi-objective optimization model attempted to combine the two goals with varying weights. Because the model is a nonlinear mixed integer program, it cannot ensure every combination had a feasible solution. The single objective model is still the best choice if decision makers only choose to make the minimum ADA standard improvements.

These two optimization models have different applicability. Based on the Broward County bus stop accessibility inventory, nearly half of the bus stops did not meet minimum ADA requirements; some of them only need a minor investment to meet the minimum ADA requirements. Meeting the minimum ADA requirements should be the priority (rather than making the investment to meet the universal design standard) due to the limited County budget. Therefore, the single objective model that aims to meet the minimum ADA standard was more suitable for Broward County. On the other hand, if a large number of the bus stops for a transit agency were qualified under the minimum ADA standard, that agency might be able to improve the accessibility of bus stop at the higher service level standard. The second model that aims to satisfy two objectives would thusly be a better choice.

The sensitivity analysis performed in this research shows that the optimization models are reasonable. The budget sensitivity analysis illustrated how the model was more efficient when the budget was lower. As the transit agency presses in making ADA improvements to the bus stops, the number of selected bus stops will decrease each year. Factor sensitivity analysis was used to inspect how the changes in the weight value for the different factors affect the optimization model. The model output showed that the weighted curve changed smoothly for each factor. The changes in the model output were controlled throughout a reasonable area when the ratio of each factor changed. Compared to the usual basis on which bus stops are slated for improvement (staff experience or requests from elected officials), this decision tool provides a more reasonable platform on which to make improvement suggestions.

7.3. Recommendations

The following recommendations are made to further improve the results from the two optimization models developed in this research:

1. The population with disabilities in this research was disaggregated in terms of the census blockgroup level, and their transportation to work was at the Traffic Analysis Zone (TAZ) level. These gross analysis zones will impair the reliability of final optimization model. If data are available at such level as household parcels, future efforts should be made to use such data rather than at the census blockgroup or TAZ level, in order to obtain more precise distance calculation between a trip origin (or destination) and the nearest bus stop.

2. The distance decay model illustrates that the probability of demand falls as walking distance increases. In this model, intercept parameter a and slope parameter b were analyzed based on the general population. The probability curve of demand for persons with disabilities should fall more dramatically based on walking distance than for ambulatory people. More effort can be made to adjust the two parameters, or develop a new distance decay model specifically designed for populations with disabilities.

3. In this research, the budget for shelter improvement was based on the bus stop ADA improvement budget. Unfortunately, the budget for shelter improvement came from other sources—the transit agency as well as advertisement venders. Shelter improvements directly relate to the service level for riders with disabilities. Further study may focus on how to combine among the different shelter improvement budget sources in order to provide better services for riders with disabilties.

4. Sidewalk improvements are very costly. Although the basic cost estimation in this research was based on the nearest intersections, many other factors were not taken into consideration including obstacles, joining with the other sidewalk or facilities, and the work hours needed for construction. Future efforts can be made to identify additional variables to better estimate sidewalk distance and construction cost.

5. In this research, all bus stop construction was based on single bus stop or a group of bus stops. Transit agencies usually prefer bus stop improvement along a specific route or a street. The optimization models developed in this research can be ehanced to consider improvements based on different construction requests, including routes.

REFERENCES

1. Broward County Transit, Broward County Transit Development Plan, http://www.broward.org/transportationplanning/tpi02601.pdf, 2005.

2. Chakhar, S., and V. Mousseau, "Spatial Multicriteria Decision Making," *Encyclopedia of Geographical Information Science*, Springer, 2007.

3. Church, R. L., and J. R. Marston, "Measuring Accessibility for People with a Disability," *Geographical Analysis*, 35(1), 2003, pp. 83-96.

4. Church, R., and C. ReVelle, "The Maximal Covering Location Problem," *Papers of the Regional Science Association 32*, 1974, pp. 101-118.

5. Collia, D. V., J. Sharp, and L. Giesbrecht, "The 2001 National Household Travel Survey: A Look into the Travel Patterns of Older Americans," *Journal of Safety Research*, 34, 2003, pp. 461-470.

6. Department of Justice, "Code of Federal Regulations: ADA Standards for Accessible Design," Washington DC, 1994.

7. Easter Seals Project ACTION, "Toolkit for Bus Stop Accessibility and Safety Assessment," Washington, DC, 2005.

8. ESRI, "ArcGIS 9 – Using ArcGIS' Spatial Analyst," http://downloads.esri.com/support/documentation/ao_/776Using_Spatial_Analyst.pdf, 2007

9. ESRI, "ArcIMS 9 – Customizing ArcIMS—Using the ActiveX Connector," http://arsc.arid.arizona.edu/resources/web_dev/activex_connector/Customizing_ActiveX.pdf, 2002.

10. Federal Transit Administration (FTA), "Accessibility Handbook for Transit Facilities," Malvern, PA, 1992.

11. Florida Planning and Development Lab, "Accessing Transit: Design Handbook for Florida Bus Passenger Facilities," Florida State University, Tallahassee, FL, 2004.

12. Florida Planning and Development Lab, "From Bus Shelters to Transit Oriented Development: a Literature Review of Bus Passenger Facility Planning, Siting, and Design," Florida State University, Tallahassee, FL, 2004.

13. GAMS Development Corporation,"GAMS - A User's Guide," http://www.gams.com/docs/gams/GAMSUsersGuide.pdf, 2007.

14. Kimpel, T. J., K. J. Dueker, and M. El-Geneidy, "Using GIS to Measure the Effect of Overlapping Service Areas on Passenger Boardings at Bus Stops," *URISA Journal*, Vol. 19, No.1, 2007.

15. Law, P., and B. D. Taylor, "Shelter from the Storm: Optimizing the Distribution of Bus Stop Shelters in Los Angeles," *Transportation Research Record 1753*, National Research Council, Washington, DC, 2001, pp. 79-85.

16. Lehman Center for Transportation Research, "ATSIM User's Guide Version 3.0," Florida International University, Miami, FL, 2007.

17. Malczewski, J., *GIS and Multicriteria Decision Analysis,* John Wiley & Sons, Inc., New York, 1999.

18. Moldovanyi, A., "GIS and Multi-Criteria Decision Making to Determine Marketability of Pay Pond Businesses in West Virginia," *Aquaculture Forum in West Virginia University*, Morgantown, WV, 2004.

19. Murray, A. T., "A Coverage Model for Improving Public Transit System Accessibility and Expanding Access," *Annals of Operations Research*, 123, 2003, pp. 143-156.

20. National Council on Disability, "The Current State of Transportation for People with Disabilities in the United States," Washington, DC, 2004.

21. 'Olio, L. D., J. L. Moura, and A. Ibeas, "Bus Transit Accessibility for People with Reduced Mobility: The Case of Oviedo, Spain," *ITE Journal*, 125(5), 2007, pp. 28-32.

22. Roy, B., *Multicriteria Methodology for Decision Aiding,* Kluwer Academic Publishers, Dordrecht, The Netherlands, 1996.

23. Scottish Executive Transport Research Planning Group, "Improved Public Transport for Disabled People," http://www.scotland.gov.uk/Publications/2006/05/16145134/10, 2006.

24. Thill, J., *Spatial Multicriteria Decision Making and Analysis: a Geographic Information Sciences Approach,* Ashgate Publishing Ltd, Brookfield, VT, 1999.

25. Toregas, C., R. Swain, C. ReVelle, and L. Bergmen, "The Location of Emergency Service Facilities," *Operations Research 19*, 1971, pp. 1363-1373.

26. Transit Cooperative Research Program, "Guidelines for the Location and Design of Bus Stops," TCRP Report 19, Washington, DC, 1996.

27. U.S. Census Bureau, "Americans with Disabilities: 2002 Household Economic Studies," Washington, DC, 2006.

28. U.S. Department of Transportation, "Freedom to Travel," Washington, DC, 2003.

29. Zhao, F., "GIS Analysis of the Impact of Community Design on Transit Accessibility," *ASCE South Florida Section 1998 Annual Meeting*, Sanibel Island, FL, 1998.

30. Zhao, F., L. Chow, M. Li, I. Ubaka, and A. Gan. "Forecasting Transit Walk Accessibility: Regression Model Alternative to Buffer Method," *Transportation Research Record 1835*, National Research Council, Washington, DC, 2003, pp.34-41.

31. Zhu, X., and S. Liu, "An Integrated GIS Approach to Accessibility Analysis," *Transactions in GIS*, 8(1), 2004, pp. 45-62.

32. Zhu, X., S. Liu, and M. C. Yeow, "A GIS-Based Multi-Criteria Analysis Approach to Accessibility Analysis for Housing Development in Singapore," *The National Biennial Conference of the Spatial Sciences Institute*, Melbourne, 2005.

LIST OF ACRONYMS

ACTION	Accessible Community Transportation In Our Nation
ADA	Americans with Disabilities Act
ADAAG	ADA Accessibility Guidelines
AHP	Analytical Hierarchy Process
APC	Automatic Passenger Counter
API	Application Programming Interface
ATSIM	Automated Transit Stop Inventory Model
BCT	Broward County Mass Transit
BTS	Bureau of Transportation Statistics
CTPP	Census Transportation Planning Package
FGDL	Florida Geographic Data Library
FHWA	Federal Highway Administration
FTIS	Florida Transit Information System
GAMS	General Algebraic Modeling System
GIS	Geographic Information System
GPS	Global Positioning System
GUI	Graphical User Interface
LCTR	Lehman Center for Transportation Research
LINDO	Linear, INteractive, and Discrete Optimizer
LINGO	Integer programming, Linear programming, Nonlinear programming, Global Optimization
LSCP	Location Set Covering Problem
MCDM	Multicriteria Decision Making
MCLP	Maximal Covering Location Problem
NHTS	National Household Travel Survey
PDA	Personal Digital Assistant
RAD	Rapid Application Development
RV	Recreational Vehicle
TCRP	Transit Cooperative Research Program
TDP	Transit Development Plan
TIP	Transportation Improvement Program
UDD	Uniform Density of Demand
UFAS	Uniform Federal Accessibility Standards
VBA	Visual Basic for Application
XML	Extensible Markup Language

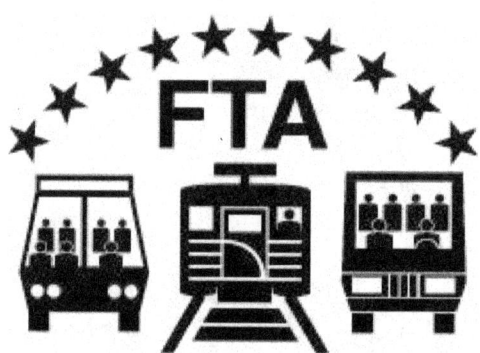

Office of Research, Demonstration, and Innovation
U.S. Department of Transportation
1200 New Jersey Avenue, SE
Washington, D.C. 20590

http://www.fta.dot.gov/research

Report No. FTA-FL-04-7104-2010.03